Before and After Loss

A Johns Hopkins Press Health Book

Before
AND
After
Loss

A NEUROLOGIST'S PERSPECTIVE
ON LOSS, GRIEF, AND OUR BRAIN

———————— • ————————

LISA M. SHULMAN, MD

JOHNS HOPKINS UNIVERSITY PRESS • BALTIMORE

© 2018 Johns Hopkins University Press
All rights reserved. Published 2018
Printed in the United States of America on acid-free paper
9 8 7 6 5 4 3

Johns Hopkins University Press
2715 North Charles Street
Baltimore, Maryland 21218
www.press.jhu.edu

Library of Congress Cataloging-in-Publication Data

Names: Shulman, Lisa M., author.
Title: Before and after loss : a neurologist's perspective on loss, grief,
    and our brain / Lisa M. Shulman.
Other titles: Johns Hopkins Press health book.
Description: Baltimore : Johns Hopkins University Press, 2018. | Series: Johns
    Hopkins Press health book | Includes bibliographical references and index.
Identifiers: LCCN 2018010712| ISBN 9781421426945 (hardcover : alk. paper) |
    ISBN 1421426943 (hardcover : alk. paper) | ISBN 9781421426952
    (paperback : alk. paper) | ISBN 1421426951 (paperback : alk. paper) |
    ISBN 9781421426969 (electronic) | ISBN 142142696X (electronic)
Subjects: LCSH: Grief. | Bereavement. | Healing. | MESH: Grief | Emotional
    Adjustment | Attitude to Death | Psychological Trauma—rehabilitation |
    Personal Narratives
Classification: LCC BF575.G7 S48 2018 | DDC 155.9/3—dc23
LC record available at https://lccn.loc.gov/2018010712

A catalog record for this book is available from the British Library.

Special discounts are available for bulk purchases of this book. For more informa-
tion, please contact Special Sales at 410-516-6936 or specialsales@press.jhu.edu.

To Bill

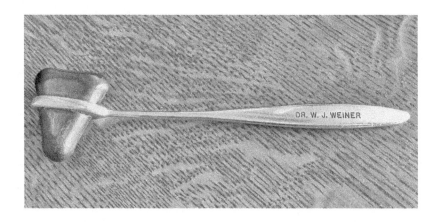

There would be no lobby into this house, and there would be no "introduction" into it or into the novel. I wanted the reader to be kidnapped, thrown ruthlessly into an alien environment as the first step into a shared experience with the book's population—just as the characters were snatched from one place to another, from any place to any other, without preparation or defense.

—Toni Morrison,
Foreword to *Beloved*

Contents

Preface

I expected grief to be unbearable sadness, but it wasn't that at all.
It was profound instability.
Losing bearings, losing identity, losing your coherent self.
Where life is distorted, spooling out in a surreal string of events.
Where sorrow is expected, and altered reality arrives.

As COMMON AS BIRTH, death is simply part of human experience. Yet we strain to comprehend life's passages—the beginning of a new life and the end of another. Addition is easier to grasp than subtraction, the tangible instead of the void. The beginning and end of life are natural, organic. Yet death and grief lie outside the mainstream, veering toward ambiguity and mystery. In these pages, we explore not only the experience but also the science and psychology of grief and loss.

In 2011, my husband and colleague, Dr. William Weiner, was diagnosed with cancer. He died seventeen months later, in December 2012. Bill and I were both neurologists—two physician-scientists confronting our own health crises. Abruptly, the tables turned as we became patients, rather than physicians. As events unfolded, the space between our previous understanding of our patients' experience and our day-to-day reality widened.

This book draws upon our personal experience with grave illness and loss to assist others confronting similar experiences. A neurologist is an expert in brain science and a keen observer of behavior, someone who understands that behavior is a reflection of function of the brain and the mind. In this book, both our professional and personal lives are brought to bear on the challenges we faced. Here, we are both the observer and the observed.

I've studied coping and adjustment to chronic illness for many years. The disorientation of grief is itself a chronic condition, an altered state where our minds strain to find order in a jumble of unfamiliar events. But knowledge about coping with life wasn't preparation for coping with death. I was ill-prepared for what was to come.

This book explores the interface between the experience of profound loss and the search for emotional restoration and healing. The experience of loss is the setting, but our main focus is the transition from grief to restoration—navigating the transition from grief to a new stage of life.

Grieving is a protective process. It's an evolutionary adaptation to help us survive in the face of emotional trauma. Although we usually envision physical trauma when we think of traumatic brain injury, here we'll focus on emotional trauma as the cause of brain injury and on its consequences for daily function. The experience of grief can overwhelm us, but understanding the science behind grief can dispel mystery and restore a sense of control. Shedding light on the psychology and science of emotional trauma places our experience in a larger context. Individually, the experience is unfamiliar and surreal, but there's comfort to be found in understanding how our brain responds and heals following traumatic loss. We'll review what is known about the effects of loss and grieving on the mind, brain, and body.

We'll also explore the self-efficacy of grieving—our sense of control during periods of grief—and steps we can take to restore confidence and control. Self-efficacy is the confidence we have in our ability to handle challenges and difficult situations. Importantly, self-efficacy improves with better knowledge, insight, and tools to manage our situation. A better sense of control helps us find a path forward. Grief is perilous. It leaves us exposed. Our experiences are personal. We'll survey the landscape of loss and healing, but in the end, the answers come from within.

Journaling is a potent tool of healing employed in these pages, with themes framed for personal reflections. From the earliest days of his diagnosis, Bill and I agreed to keep separate journals. We didn't know what was to come, but we recognized the value of our experience—the reflections of two disease specialists on the disease experience. With Bill gone, I continued writing scattered thoughts and experiences. I became aware of moments when suffering was relieved by transforming waves of emotion into words and coherent sentences. Where emotion was amorphous, words on a page were reassuringly concrete. It was months later that I recognized my healing ritual was simply *journaling*.

Journaling involves telling your story, being mindful in describing experience. Our stories contain layers of meaning to explore by giving voice to memory and emotion. Seeing the story on the page demystifies traumatic events and lessens the hold these events have on us. As we recall and unravel our experience, insight deepens and bewilderment lessens. We see things with more perspective. We think more clearly. And our interpretation deepens over time—days, months, and years later when we return to read our own words, literally making reflections on reflections.

In the early months of writing, I contemplated turning my journal into a book. As I moved into the second year without Bill, I questioned whether I had anything original to contribute and whether the time had come to look forward, not back. Yet the urge to document memories and insights had its own life. Notes scribbled by day and night piled up around me. And with time the book's purpose came into focus. The goal is less memoir, more guidebook, to shed light on common experiences of traumatic loss and how our brain responds and heals. Bill's and my experiences are found in these pages, and they are carefully chosen to deepen understanding of the experience of loss and to lay the foundation for approaches to healing.

Many memoirs of loss are available, and finding passages that affirm our experience is comforting and therapeutic. But by and large, books of this genre don't capture the distinction between the depression and the trauma of grief. And they rarely pivot from description of loss to describing the tools needed to move forward and facilitate emotional restoration. Understanding the science and psychology of grief dispels the mystery of bereavement and raises awareness of the experience of traumatic loss. The goal is to increase our sense of confidence and control for managing loss and grief.

We're united by the experience of loss. But our losses are different and our sources of comfort and support vary. Condolences and support from family and friends are important, but they can be diminished by the isolating intimacy of loss. Grief is personal, not shared. Grief is a distinctive experience that doesn't fit with other challenges. We shouldn't be surprised that we're ill equipped to handle this. Conventional approaches may not meet the complex needs of grief. We often draw strength from the unexpected while being deflated by our expectations of traditional sources of comfort.

We're on this path together. We've lost something precious—a person who anchored us, who guided us, who gave our life meaning. We may feel less than whole. With both daily routines and expectations for the future upended, life itself loses value. In these worst of times, we look for guidance on how to rebuild our lives. With time, condolence and remembrance must give way to restoration and renewal. Those we have lost expect nothing less from us.

I focused on the simple metaphor of putting one foot in front of the other each day, searching for a path to move forward instead of walking in place. It often seemed aimless and groping; only in retrospect did my hoped-for path emerge. Setbacks on this path are inevitable, and it's easy to believe that these setbacks represent personal failures rather than routine, transient experiences. Even observing our capacity to recover following setbacks may not be sufficient to dispel fear, despondence, and the sense we're letting ourselves down—especially when we stumble again. Only in retrospect do we perceive the role that disorientation and instability played.

As we grapple with loss, let's be thoughtful about healing, restoration, and growth. Let's not be satisfied with healing and restoration alone, let's strive for growth. Healing results in the survival of a coherent self after traumatic loss. Growth recasts today's insurmountable problems as tomorrow's opportunities.

> When I let go of what I am,
> I become what I might be.
> —LAO TZU

In the final weeks of Bill's life, I scarcely grasped what was happening to him, no less what was to come for me. The loss of personal identity was sudden and unexpected. And that is what this book is about: experiencing the loss of life as you know it and the search for emotional restoration.

From the earliest days, there was a need to make sense of senseless loss. That urge underlies many ambitious projects in honor of loved ones. Bill continues to inspire me to be creative, to be bold, and to tell you about our before and after life.

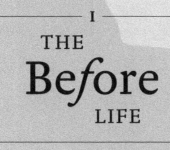

I

THE
Before
LIFE

CHAPTER 1

•

But We Will

THE WAITING ROOM IS TINY, dimly lit. White noise muffles the voices of Bill and the counselor. Seated in an oddly low chair, I wait my turn, organizing my thoughts. But as his prognosis becomes dire, clarity of thought recedes, replaced by periods of miasma. An altered state where thoughts begin, then spontaneously abort. *Our first visit to a counselor . . . today's lab results . . . is Bill ok in there? . . . tonight's dinner . . . the doctor told us . . .* Each false start enveloped by fog, each thought, just . . . pauses. Then I'm back, recalling where I am and why we're here. Ironic: the box on the side table emits white noise, like the white noise filling my head, clouding my mind. I am dimly aware of these strange patterns of thought—the incoherence, the fleeting insights. *We're dying . . . Bill and I are dying.*

I need not hear the voices to know what Bill is saying. He's straightforward and unsentimental. His words are tinged with irony. He has little capacity for introspection, much less for self-analysis. Uncommonly intuitive, he relies on instinct. Even as weak as he is, the counselor will be no match for him. He'll direct things, as he always does, getting his message across and deflecting topics along the way. His message: *I'm dying and I have little time left. You'll be speaking to Lisa. We've built a joyous life together with few attachments to others. She'll be alone. You need to watch over her.* The two sides of intimacy are palpable, the vulnerability of entwined lives.

The passage of time weighs on us, stretching and constricting the days in unfamiliar patterns. The pain will end for one of us; for the other, the pain will endure. Three losses approach: the loss of him, the loss of us, and the loss of who I am.

BILL LIVED LIFE ARTFULLY and with grace. He was more than husband, colleague, mentor, confidant. Bill made an impact on many lives and was no less than transformational in mine. Living life with wisdom, he possessed a fine balance—of power and tenderness, intensity and patience, listening and speaking out, exuberance and peaceful reflection, high expectations yet forgiveness.

The clattering of pots and pans announced a new culinary adventure. He was pickling vegetables, baking bread, heating fragrant Middle Eastern spices, assembling a comforting stew. Or planning trips to the farmers market and fairs of all types: crafts, antiques, quilts, old bottles. I see him sitting on the couch after breakfast reading the paper and planning our next adventure. My workaholic self would hesitate, then relent. I'd catch the playful look on his face when he caught me enjoying myself to the fullest. I was spurred to be his muse, for the simple reward of watching his face light up. My reward was relishing his joy—our life was vibrant, dynamic, vital. From the tranquility of our home, to collegial collaboration, to the thrill of exotic travel, it was in a word, sublime.

I thrilled to the way his face lit up when our eyes met;
the way he reached into his pocket for special gifts in the most
    ordinary of times;
the way he was stirred by matters of principle;
his ravenous appetite for life—diving in and taking big gulps;
his steady encouragement to spread my wings: Of course
    you'll do it;
the way his body relaxed preparing drinks at the end of the day;
and the way he leaned in close to my ear to whisper, I want to be
    alone with you,
like the wistful expression in Renoir's Dance at Bougival, *that*
    moment when the world pauses.

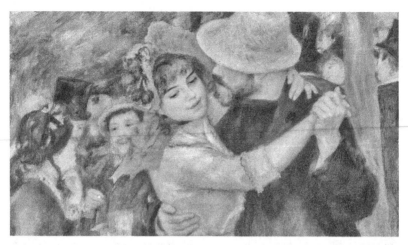

Pierre-Auguste Renoir's *Dance at Bougival* (detail). PHOTOGRAPH © 2018 MUSEUM OF FINE ARTS, BOSTON

WE WERE SIPPING COFFEE on a bright summer morning full of promise, starting our Maine vacation, when we learned Bill was dying. It all began suddenly—the beginning of the end. Bill described lower back pain as people do. I was making coffee when an unsettling thought arrived. It was the first morning I could recall arriving in the kitchen before Bill. I found him in the bedroom, his face etched in apprehension and pain. *Let's take care of this today so we can enjoy the rest of our vacation.*

We called a local neurologist colleague who expedited our visit that morning. His exam was reassuring and unrevealing. An MRI (magnetic resonance imaging) scan—just to be thorough. In the hospital waiting room, I turned pages of outdated magazines. It all seemed so ordinary until I saw the neurologist coming toward me. I knew in that first glance we were in trouble.

It turned out I knew a lot more about living than dying. In my work, I studied quality of life, unaware I knew little about quality of death, and even less about quality of life after death.

Bill was dying, and neither of us found shelter in hope of another outcome. Among the most difficult things during this most difficult time was how intimacy was a barrier to communication. Intimacy can be a barrier when death approaches. It's a time when an abundance of joy becomes an abundance of despair. When awareness of the loss of him and the loss of us coalesce in an ocean of desolation. When thoughts of death echo and reverberate between us, rising to a painful chord that neither of us could bear. We recognize our days are numbered and quietly witness our demise. Death tears us apart from people closest to us, from people we bond with in ways that render us less than whole without them.

We couldn't look into each other's eyes to acknowledge our end. *Bill, we're going through a terrible time; maybe it's more than we can handle alone. We confide in one another. But now, we're stumbling because we care too deeply for each other. It's too painful for us—maybe we need to speak to someone else.* Without hesitation, Bill agreed . . . because he knew I needed it. I told myself it was important for us, but now I see: it was for me.

> Dying, however, is lonely, the loneliest event of life.
> Dying not only separates you from others but also
> exposes you to a second, even more frightening form
> of loneliness: separation from the world itself.
> —IRVIN D. YALOM, *Staring at the Sun:*
> *Overcoming the Terror of Death*

For Bill, incapacity was unendurable. I focused on ways to support his instincts, to respect his dignity, to maintain our balance. Confronting the loss of him, the loss of us, I strained to maintain focus. The events, the moments in time, when Bill and I saw what we were up against accumulated as we shifted from stress to trauma to survival. And in Bill's final months, my failure to make things better, to alleviate suffering, to bring him peace, was unbearable.

Illness increasingly defined our world. At times, we were united against the enormity of what we faced. At other times illness was a rising barrier between us, an alien line where we found ourselves on opposite sides, where disease was a terrible burden that could not be shared.

Illness dismantled our lives, despite our best efforts to substitute, to rebuild, to compensate, to be resourceful. As physicians, we witnessed how illness erodes spirit as layers of personhood are stripped away. And we watched how the balance and reciprocity of relationships were distorted by disability. Life's events continuously challenged this dynamic, requiring recurrent modulation of our roles. But the decline of grave illness is not like other events: it's a series of defining moments where import rises as capacity declines. Mutuality compounded each event as we experienced every moment through each other's eyes and through our own. Here, intimacy sowed the seeds of emotional trauma.

We harbored no delusions after a year of failed treatments. On a rare day home from the hospital, I looked at Bill and thought about the value of giving voice to our deepest thoughts. The ease and intimacy that came naturally to us faltered in our time of need. While there was still time, I wanted to be guided by his thoughts and instincts. I tried to draw him out, and failed again. In earlier months, his responses were cryptic, but also revealing. One evening after a long hospital day, we quietly prepared dinner side by side. *But you told me we would grow old together,* I said. And he replied, *But we will.*

In the final weeks, there was his quiet determination to accept what could not be changed. Bill's essence was caring and doing for others. The energy he brought to this task was matched by his disregard for self-analysis. If he could not be who he was, life held little value. In these days of great import, I was pulled in different directions: to help him feel safe and at peace; to suppress my desperation for intimacy; to support his need for quiet separation. Our lives had aligned effortlessly, but in these final weeks our paths parted. We were not traveling to the same place. *But we will,* he said. *I will always be with you, but not in the way we imagined.*

We call it grief. But grief is just the surface of a yawning canyon of loss. You slip over the edge and tumble down without precedent to guide or handholds to grasp. Witnessing birth—or death—is life altering, sacred. We can't fathom the first breath of a newborn, no less the last breath of the person we travel through life with.

Loss is not a single event, it's a series of unspeakable events. Yet we look deceptively the same, concealing the wounds of emotional trauma—raw, weeping wounds. The derivation of the word grief is "to burden," as if people experiencing grief are weighed down by external troubles. But grief is a consuming internal process. The injury is hidden, even from us.

Witnessing decline, watching the loss of a soul—the soul you share and know better than all others—is walking to the very edge of the end of life and peeking, even taking a small step, over the side. The sense you exist partly on this other side is a profound state, incompatible with day-to-day life. The daily routines—the chit-chat, the pleasantries, the weather, the office gossip . . . expending energy to simply fit into this world while having one foot in the other.

Imperceptibly, the mind adapts to this altered state, becoming a filter that tempers disorientation and pain. The subconscious senses and sets the threshold, sorting what gets through to maintain equilibrium. Bit by bit, insight is diminished, perspective is distorted. Attention is paid to what's perceived; the fragmentation of reality isn't apparent. With illness and decline, the balance of responsibility and decision-making shifts. The weight of managing our lives and making grave decisions accelerates, demanding partitioning of thinking from feeling. Yet in the worst of times, priorities are attended to, and externally, we appear to be holding up well . . . to be normal.

THE WAITING ROOM DOOR OPENS and Bill appears. He stares at me, pale and stricken. Leaning heavily on his walking stick, he moves across the room with unnatural wooden strides. I babble—*Are you ok? . . . Do you need anything? . . . Are you sure?*—walking the vanishing line between concern and overprotection. Anxiety chips away at finesse and fear creeps into my voice. I hesitate. Is it safe to leave him? He nods and points to the door. As I walk into the office, I am filled with dread: *We're moving in opposite directions.*

The counselor's face echoes Bill's expression—as if pain permeates everything around us. My mind's white noise drowns out all memory of why I'm here. My mind is blank. I envision Bill waiting outside. *What was I thinking? There's nothing to say, there are no words.* We stare at each other in silence. Bleakness. Desolation. *What is there to say? Why did I suggest this?*

My thoughts are inaccessible—like a mind wrapped in thick gauze.

Underneath the gauze—a gaping wound.

Too horrible to look at—too painful to bear.

And then the silence is broken . . .

I am in mortal danger.

I hear somebody say that.

I think . . . that is me.

CHAPTER 2

◆

We Are Sick

IT WAS ONLY ME and a young man outside the MRI suite. I was learning a lot about the ups and downs of his multiple sclerosis, while trying to return to a magazine. Picking up the vibe, he described his surprise that Michael J. Fox had turned 50 and had Parkinson's disease, the cover story of the *Good Housekeeping* magazine on my lap. The magazine interview with Fox caught my attention—when asked how he and his wife cope with Parkinson's, he described two techniques he had learned as an actor: *know what* and *as if*. Even though the actor knows how the story ends, he must act like he doesn't *know what* will happen. Instead, the actor behaves *as if* he's in the moment. With a serious diagnosis, it's best to live life without certainty you *know what's* ahead, and to live *as if* in the moment. I chewed on thoughts of how this could be useful to our patients when I saw the neurologist and radiologist approaching. One glance told it all: *We're in trouble.*

There were bony lesions damaging Bill's spine at many levels. *It doesn't look good . . . cancer.* I interrupted as the radiologist listed possible diagnoses: *Does Bill know?* I found him still in the scanner waiting for additional scans, and he knew. He lay on the narrow platform with a strap across his forehead. We looked into each other's eyes. Grief was born in those first moments.

As the spine images flashed on the screen in front of us, Bill's voice was thick with emotion: *That's just great.* The radiologist explained that the likely diagnosis was metastatic cancer, most likely lung, colon, or prostate. There were many bony lesions, one particularly nasty one in Bill's lower back, the source of his back pain. Bill said, *How about multiple myeloma?*—a blood cancer that invades the bone. We stared at the dark blotches staining the smooth white bone of the spine, leaving destruction in its wake in the most painful bony segment and wantonly invading others. Spine MRI images, not at all unfamiliar to neurologists. We quietly appraised the enemy: aggressive, invasive, heartless.

We drove away from the hospital in stunned silence. The plan was to shop for halibut, avocados, and lime for fish tacos to welcome arriving family, but Bill was driving back to our vacation home. I was experiencing the first sense of being in unfamiliar terrain, struggling to shunt aside emotion and focus on what Bill needed now, what to do, what to say. *Let's stop at the harbor.* We walked to a favorite bench at the edge of Rockport Harbor—a beautiful spot. As I hugged and kissed Bill, an elderly man stopped by to kid him: *If she's bothering you, just let me know.* We watched the man and his wife slowly walk to the next bench to unwrap their dinner for a picnic—a simple, lovely moment. We had the same thought: *Was this still in our future?* On that bench, I told Bill all about *know what* and *as if.* He mulled it over and firmly said, *Ok, I'm going with that.* We used those phrases as our mantra in the difficult days to come.

But that night as we lay in bed, Bill's whole body began to shake uncontrollably. Minutes passed as I held him tightly until we fell asleep. We awakened later to hold each other and cry silently into the night.

Two days later we were back on the road, returning home to Baltimore. Our plans for peaceful weeks in Maine lingered as our minds filled with the long road ahead—diagnosis and treatment. Bill loved a drive on the open road. As we headed onto the thruway we passed a road sign: "Rockport to Denver 2,154 miles, Rockport to Los Angeles 3,160 miles . . . " Bill said, *How about this: let's take the turn toward*

Denver and just keep going. We looked at each other. It sounded good
then and it sounds good now. The urge to be free, to flee from the
medical labyrinth, was powerful. The car slowed as we gazed at that
exit ramp passing by.

A full day of tests to look for cancer throughout the body, followed
by the oncologist's verdict. All of Bill's organs were normal; only his
bones were affected. The diagnosis: blood cancer. Multiple myeloma,
as Bill suspected when we first saw the spine images. The oncologist's
summation: *It's not trivial, but better than it could have been.* We
stopped for coffee and marveled how we were buoyed by this news . . .
cancer—but there was reason for hope.

....

BILL'S JOURNAL

*This last week has been tumultuous—we went from settling into
our work/vacation home overlooking Rockport Harbor to facing
serious illness. Since about age 30, I've been in the business of
delivering life-altering news to my patients—I thought I had
come to understand the impact of the news I delivered, but the
phrase "turning the world upside down" is never fully understood
until you're on the receiving end—the radiologist walking into
the room during the MRI to say I need more images—Why?—
Looks like metastatic cancer—How can that be?—Lisa and I
were convinced this was just a common back problem. When we
saw the scan, I felt nothing but dread and worry about myself
and Lisa. So, Friday 8/5 changed from relaxing and preparing
menus for arriving family, to making calls to the director of the
cancer center and preparing to leave Maine to seek diagnosis
and treatment in Baltimore. Multiple days and tests later the
diagnosis is multiple myeloma—rather serious but in light of
what we saw on the initial scan and the radiologist's impression,
this was definitely a "better" diagnosis.*

....

As physicians, describing prognosis and treatment options to newly
diagnosed patients was familiar territory: giving enough information,

but not too much; finding the right tone and level of complexity; treading the line between evidence and uncertainty. And that is the hard truth in medicine. There isn't a single correct approach to treating disease; there are always unanswered questions. The data you need isn't available when you need it. The myeloma specialist was clear, concise, realistic, and hopeful—he struck that balance of honesty and hope that we, too, sought with our patients. *Are we going to be ok?* The treatment, response, and side effects would unfold, but *our ability to be ok*—to be resilient, flexible, and resourceful, to simply remain who we were—was in our own hands.

IT'S FRIDAY EVENING, the weekly Sabbath day of rest, when we light candles at sundown and pause to mark the moment, to be mindful of our life and family. I hesitate as an unfamiliar, bitter taste of anger rises. But Bill calmly takes the silver candlesticks out and prepares two glasses of wine. I do it for him . . . and for us.

....

BILL'S JOURNAL

I'm thinking about lighting Shabbat candles in our beautiful home and then dancing with Lisa—Why light the candles? What does it mean? Recently with the advent of the diagnosis, it's been more difficult to light the candles in peace, particularly for Lisa. When we light candles and say the blessing of the lights together, we're making a small amount of time more precious to spend together. Things can't always be exactly as we wish but certain rituals remain—I still view lighting the candles and saying the blessing of the lights together as special moments of reflection, love, quiet, and peace.

....

Bill lives in the moment while maintaining a long and balanced perspective. He has few inner demons, accepting the rhythm of life with grace. Yet he's also a man of strong ideas, high passion, and strong tastes. He's sensitive and romantic: a brown paper bag reveals champagne, crystal flutes, and strawberries on my birthday, and a note tucked into my purse during difficult times reads, *I miss you. Things will go well! I love you.* We're struggling to find a new balance. Bill's default—a healthy combination of optimism, denial, and living in the moment—is serving him well.

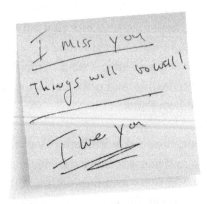

A note from
Bill to Lisa

I FLOW ALONG THE CURRENTS of Bill's instincts as we begin chemotherapy. We focus on the proactive part of it: killing myeloma cells, fighting back against this invasion in our life. We don't want these poisons, but the cancer infusion suite isn't what we expected; the atmosphere is upbeat and compassionate, with a quiet camaraderie among the patients and families. There's a rhythm to the process: two weeks of chemotherapy followed by a week off for "staging." The first twenty-four hours after, Bill feels better, but forty-eight hours later he's not himself. Frequent trips to the pharmacy to find the right antidotes.

....

BILL'S JOURNAL

Day #1 of treatment—over the weekend I thought a lot about writing about how I was feeling and whether it will be the last time I felt "normal" but then I decided it's better to write an entry after the day in the infusion center. I and Lisa view treatment as the start of reclaiming our lives and work—the first step of a journey back to us. So it's not really Day #1 but a continuum of our joyous journey together.

....

It's only a week later that more bad news arrives. Genetic tests were performed on the bone marrow cells for information on individual prognosis. There is a mutation, an extra copy of a chromosome, and it's not good news. The chances for remission and for a long remission are not good. As we watch the chemotherapy infusion drip into Bill's arm, this news crushes our hopes for a long reprieve. The hospital curtains are pulled around us, to give us time alone to absorb this before rejoining our colleagues in cancer.

I'm emotional while Bill is calm. He says we probably weren't listening well the first week. Things are now sinking in, but Bill says he's still optimistic. He will do better than average. He will be the outlier. We will be ok. He asks, *What are you thinking about?* I say, *I want to grow old together.* Bill says many times that day, *We will grow old together.*

The next day at chemotherapy, the hospital shakes and rattles for a minute. An unprecedented 5.9 earthquake has rocked most of the eastern seaboard. And four days later, Hurricane Irene passes through. Strange things are happening.

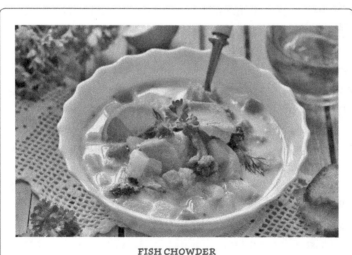

FISH CHOWDER
August 2011
A wonderful dinner following chemotherapy today. Bill loves fish chowder. We use salmon, halibut, tuna, and extra veggies—carrots and fennel.
Bill & Lisa

WITH THE END OF SUMMER, we return to the office. We're feeling our way through this. Bill continues with chemotherapy infusions in the cancer center just across from our office. We strive to integrate the expected and unexpected into our daily lives. Who to tell; how to tell what's going on. Bill is the chair of the Department of Neurology. His welfare has consequences for many. Our fragile balance is perturbed by reactions of staff and colleagues—a process that reverberates endlessly as symptoms become apparent and the prognosis worsens. In real time, we cope with symptoms, treatments, side effects, and the needs of family, friends, and colleagues. People care about Bill; they care about us—it's important to not be alone with this. But it's difficult to see the reflection of our fear in the faces of others. It's difficult to find words to describe how we're doing, how things are going. It's draining and sustaining all at once.

We've crossed the line from the world of the healthy to the sick: the dimension we've spent our lives peering at, studying, describing in all its facets, but which is unknowable to outsiders. We're stalked by fear that life will never return to normal, that our known life is lost.

THE SECOND CYCLE of chemotherapy is over, and Bill continues to do well. The main side effect is fatigue, requiring periodic naps in his office. I'm not comfortable caring for patients with Bill in the cancer infusion suite down the block, but he insists I do so. On these days, he sends regular text messages describing his progress to allay my anxiety and guilt for not being by his side: *IV is in . . . Waiting for lab results . . . Infusion underway . . .* and hours later, *Almost done.* It's odd to care for patients without Bill seeing patients in the next exam room. Our colleagues honor Bill's privacy and try to act normal. I'm shaky and uncertain—hovering between isolation and reaching out. I ask Bill, *What should I say?* Even in the worst of times, Bill doesn't pause: *There are no secrets—just tell the truth.*

In a twist of fate and foreshadowing, the previous chair of neurology died of myeloma just weeks after Bill was diagnosed. The former chair had recruited us to the University of Maryland and was a cherished friend. Two weeks before Bill's diagnosis, Bill was caring for this colleague when he was hospitalized with neurologic complications.

Bill's premonition of his own diagnosis at first glance at his MRI arose from his recent experience with these scans. As our former chair's condition became grave, departmental colleagues were shaken and hesitant to tell Bill since he was receiving chemotherapy for the same condition. Before dinner one evening, I told Bill the more we live this new life, the more apparent it is how things have changed for both of us: we have cancer. Then I explained, sobbing in Bill's arms, that I'd learned our colleague was in his final days. Bill already knew but had been avoiding telling me. He prepared two shots of bourbon, saying, *Here's to a great man*. After clinking glasses, we returned to quietly preparing dinner side by side and contemplating our fate.

Bill was one of three speakers at our friend's memorial service. He spoke without notes from the carved podium of the Lutheran chapel, mixing reminiscences of our colleague with flashes of humor. Few attendees knew that Bill shared more than the experience of the chairmanship. During the final hymn, Bill's voice caught, thick with emotion. It's a complex dance, being both doctor and patient.

When we return to see the oncologist to learn the results of the first round of chemotherapy, the doctor says, *You couldn't have done any better*. Bill needs this wonderful news. The back pain is nearly gone. He is moving almost normally and has stopped wearing the brace to support his lower back. Bill says, *I told you—we will grow old together*. At times we luxuriate in our simple, normal routines, and then there are other times when the days seem like a delusion—where the ground shifts, but we go on as if we haven't noticed. The day-to-day experience of grave illness can be both valiant and banal. Life's uncertainty brings everything into sharp relief. Yet the need to preserve hope results in visions of happy endings—no less for medical professionals like us.

I DON'T KNOW HOW MUCH to say to Bill and how much to keep in; I believe he feels the same. At the end of the day, we've built this beautiful, intimate relationship: we are each other's confidant. We struggle to find meaningful ways to speak about Bill's cancer, but communication is smothered by the high stakes of daily existence.

The twists and turns of our new life are steadied by the natural rhythm of the lives of our children and grandchildren: new milestones, weighty career decisions, and two new babies on their way. Before heading to bed one evening, Bill's voice cracks as he describes his daughter's request to name her new baby after him. In Judaism, children are generally named for family members who are gone, but it's permissible if a living relative agrees. It's an unexpected question, beautiful and haunting. With the baby due in a month, Bill gives this serious thought and decides against it. These are times when hope is the most basic of needs, and superstition as important as science.

IN JUDAISM, the holy day of Rosh Hashanah is the Day of Judgment, when God judges our fate for the coming year. Yom Kippur, which takes place ten days later, is a day of atonement and remembrance when this judgment is sealed. As the prayer says, *On Rosh Hashanah it is inscribed and on the fast day of Yom Kippur it is sealed . . . who shall live and who shall die.* As we listened to the traditional blowing of the shofar (ram's horn) and dipped apple in honey for "a good sweet year," we acknowledged the layers of meaning that infused our lives this year.

With chemotherapy ending, we faced the decision of stem cell transplantation. Bill leaned towards the transplant at first and was then reconsidering. Understandable—how difficult to take the risks of transplantation just when he was feeling better. A second opinion supported our oncologist's recommendation to proceed: the consultant described hundreds of successful transplants. We were uplifted by renewed encouragement and clarity. Illness calls upon us to make grave decisions. As we confronted our own, decades of experience guiding others didn't guide us. Vulnerable and exposed, not unlike our patients listening to our words, we sought to read between the lines, to scrutinize the sincerity of our physicians' words and expressions, to put our lives in their hands. As a teacher and mentor, Bill emphasized the importance of leaving patients with hope. In those moments, we learned the power and lure of hope to sustain us through the most challenging of times. As we walked out of the consultant's exam room, Bill leaned close: *I guess you're stuck with me.*

FOLLOWING FAMILY TRADITION, we rented a large house in the Hudson River Valley for Thanksgiving. With the aftereffects of chemotherapy lingering, Bill's energy wasn't what it had been, but we savored the anticipation and preparation. We planned menus weeks in advance, poring over recipes and developing a massive shopping list. We reveled in the drive North—our first trip since the fateful departure from Maine the previous summer. The house, set on acres of rolling hills, was welcoming and cozy, with a wraparound porch, a pond out front, a gazebo, and even a trampoline for the grandchildren. Best of all, it had a kitchen with enough room for everyone to prepare their assigned Thanksgiving dish together.

It was a second marriage for both of us. We each had two grown children from previous marriages and several growing families among them. As we readied the house for arriving family, there was one hitch: Bill's daughter was two weeks beyond her due date. We hoped that labor would begin in time for her to join us. Not only the baby was late, but the specially ordered organic, kosher, free-range turkey hadn't arrived. So, the Wednesday morning before Thanksgiving, we waited for news from labor and delivery (and from FedEx). The baby and turkey arrived within minutes of each other. Mazel tov, Bill, on the arrival of a grandson, 8 pounds 13 ounces—and the turkey (twice as big), which arrived moments later. At the Thanksgiving table, we toasted the newborn's arrival, bearing witness to the circle of life. It was on Thanksgiving, just one year before, that my mother died. This Thanksgiving, we welcomed a new life. In between these monumental events, cancer came into our lives.

More cycles of chemotherapy. With each passing week, the side effects accumulated—fatigue, queasiness, and nagging discomfort that Bill described as cardboard over his feet. With the cancer in remission and the stem cell transplant in the planning stages, we found a week to vacation in San Francisco and Big Sur. Surrounded by natural beauty, our plan was for emotional and physical healing, but as the week progressed, Bill's energy and mobility declined. He needed more and more rest stops as we walked through Muir Woods, and as we began touring Hearst Castle, severe leg pain overwhelmed him—he could no longer walk. We abruptly returned home, where tests showed damaged bony segments of the lower spine compressing nerves. Bill was in the operating room for back surgery shortly after. As I sat in the surgical waiting room, I thought this unexpected turn of events was a consequence of the original damage to the spine. I wasn't prepared for the surgeon's report: *The cancer is actively spreading.* In moments like these, beyond the shock of terrible news, I felt uneasy talking to the surgeon about Bill without him present, while he lay in recovery. Confronting our problems alone was so alien; it felt like betrayal. And thus began the cycle of dreaded treatments and dashed hopes, where we learned we were up against no ordinary enemy—but an enemy more resourceful than everything we had.

THE CANCER'S AGGRESSIVENESS required more aggressive approaches: the date of stem cell transplantation was moved up, and the intensity of chemotherapy was increased. As we approached this first transplant, the oncologist described the need to plan for a second stem cell transplantation to follow. The treatments and procedures became

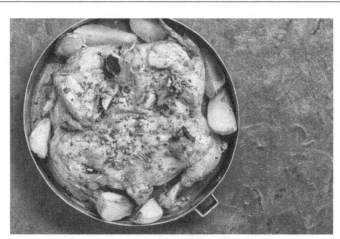

CHICKEN IN A POT
December 31, 2011
New Year's Eve. Following caviar, blinis, and champagne, we enjoyed this elegant dish. A therapeutic meal for Bill's recovery from back surgery.
Bill & Lisa

a blur: long days in the hospital, hours in waiting rooms, hospital admissions, all in an effort to suppress the cancer and optimize Bill's readiness for the stem cell transplant.

....

BILL'S JOURNAL

Lisa and I are still trying to develop better communication to talk about this situation—she feels I'm withdrawn and she feels isolated and alone—she is correct, I tend to withdraw into myself when faced with difficult emotional situations—a lifelong habit that probably started when I was young, dealing with serious illness in both parents—always feeling I should be the strong one and shoulder the burden but carry on—in other words, show no emotion and "act" normal—not an easy habit to break—now I have to try harder to communicate more with Lisa. Incidentally, I'm now BALD.

....

After one of the procedures, Bill looked reassuringly comfortable in the recovery area, although two new tubes jutted out from his chest in addition to the two tubes protruding from his arm. We were enjoying a light dinner back home when the new catheter site in the chest began seeping lots of blood-tinged fluid, loosening the dressing. I examined the site, cleaned it, and reinforced the dressing—how do people with no training handle this stuff? And how about people who live alone—how do they manage? Another evening, Bill slumped over the dinner table in a brief loss of consciousness. And another night, Bill woke at 2:00 a.m. with throbbing pain in the neck, back, and shoulders. Was this pain related to recent Neupogen injections to stimulate white blood cell production, or something else? With his blood counts so low, many alternatives came to mind: infection such as meningitis, since his immune system was weakened, or bleeding in the spinal cord or brain associated with low platelets. Temperature was normal. He was reassuringly alert and fully oriented. There was no stiff neck (seen in meningitis) but signs of inflammation could be obscured by a poor immune response. Should I call the emergency oncology number?

Should we go to the emergency department? I Googled "Neupogen back pain." The authoritative websites we tell patients to rely on weren't helpful, but the patient blogs were right on target with descriptions of bone pain that took the words right out of Bill's mouth. In our day jobs, we advised our patients to be wary of unauthoritative websites, but here, patient experience was invaluable.

Cancer relentlessly invaded our lives. How do we preserve beauty and balance? How to prevent fear and interminable time in the hospital from wearing us down? We were learning how medical environments erode confidence and optimism; how they trigger helplessness and isolation, untethered from work, from family, from community; how medical specialization fosters unease and the sense of being tossed from one group to another. Ten years ago, Bill had open heart surgery—a heart valve replacement. This was harrowing, but an altogether different experience. There was more optimism and a sense that with luck, we'd put that difficult time behind us. But this time we

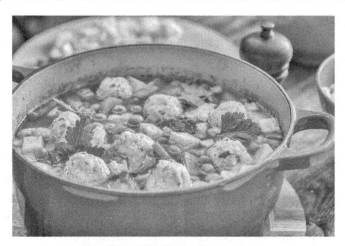

PARSNIP DUMPLINGS IN BROTH
January 2012
A very special treat—Bill's son-in-law and grandson prepared this
dinner for Bill to enjoy in the hospital. He's receiving intensive
chemotherapy, but savored the nourishing soup. As I heated the soup
in the hospital kitchen, the nurses asked, What smells so good?
The dumplings melt in your mouth—thank you!
Bill & Lisa

yearned for a reprieve, not an escape—not a return to what we had. Now we were trapped in unwanted roles as patient and caregiver, watching from the inside what we had routinely observed from the outside.

We didn't anticipate how a weak immune system fosters social isolation. There's what you feel well enough to do and then, what is safe to do. Simple pleasures hold risks of infection, like visiting small grandchildren or being out and about in a crowd. So much time in the hospital, cut off from normal life. The waiting time—mind numbing, impersonal. The setting fosters passivity, helplessness, fear . . . the *opposite* of what we try to achieve in managing disease. Patients and families are immobile, seated for hours at a time. The inactivity is debilitating, detrimental to physical and emotional health.

What we needed was an environment that reduced stress and fostered a sense of serenity and empowerment. As doctors, we asked ourselves, *Can we do better?* Here's our list of ideas, scribbled during those long days.

To Improve the Setting: More comfortable chairs, individual video monitors, computer access, relaxing music, reliable information on waiting time, and refreshments.

To Engage the Mind: Access to stimulating magazines and books, iPods with a range of podcasts (health, politics, comedy), talks and discussion groups on pertinent topics (diet, exercise, stress management, managing medications, communicating with nurses and doctors).

To Promote Activity: Encourage stretching in place and chair yoga.

To Foster Networking: Honor the experience of patients and families by conducting surveys on important topics and sharing results with the patient community.

Some of these ideas sprang from our best experiences. When we traveled to Dana-Farber Cancer Institute for Bill's consult, refreshments were available in the waiting room and volunteers offered books from a cart, then lingered to chat and pass the time with us. At the University of Maryland Medical Center surgical waiting room, my distress during Bill's back surgery was eased by a cellist's live performance. And in the Cleveland Clinic waiting room when Bill had his heart surgery, families received pagers providing progress updates, while classes oriented anxious relatives on what to expect when the patient returns to the recovery room.

This e-mail message is sent to you at the request of Dr. Weiner.

Good Morning,

  In August 2011, I was diagnosed with multiple myeloma—I have been undergoing induction chemotherapy and have had excellent results and I am now in remission—the next treatment step is an autologous bone marrow transplant which I will undergo in the coming weeks.

  The department has done extremely well based on the hard work of all our faculty and I know that all of you will continue to carry out your work in the same fine form until I return.

  Bill

William J. Weiner, MD
Professor and Chair
Department of Neurology

Six months after Bill's diagnosis, we entered the airlock door of the Bone Marrow (stem cell) Transplant Unit. In multiple myeloma, the bone marrow is the source of the cancerous cells. During the transplant, strong chemotherapy is used to wipe out the normal bone marrow. Since the bone marrow produces all our blood cells, including the white cells we depend upon for the immune response, transplant patients are at very high risk for infection. The bone marrow also produces the red blood cells we rely on to deliver oxygen and the platelets that are vital for blood clotting. The strategy is to wipe the slate clean and then deliver stem cells to the bone marrow for a fresh start—like rebooting the whole system. Neupogen, the cause of that previous night of neck and back pain, was used to stimulate Bill's bone marrow to produce fresh stem cells that were "harvested" for the stem cell transplant. Bill and I had visited the Bone Marrow Transplant Unit before, but as neurologists consulting on patients with serious complications.

Soon after arrival, Bill received an intravenous infusion of a strong toxin that brought bone marrow cell production to a halt over the next few days. The side effects began almost immediately: nausea, complete loss of appetite, and sleepiness. I asked, *What would happen if you don't follow the toxin with the stem cell transplant?* The oncologist responded, *He would die.* Once the toxin was given, followed by the infusion of Bill's own stem cells, the clock was ticking for two weeks while his bone marrow production ceased and we waited for the stem cells to "take root" (engraft) and nudge the blood counts upward again. Family and I waited at the bedside, covered from head to toe: mask, hat, gown, gloves. At times, he was so pale and still that I moved close just to see him breathing.

A blood cell count calendar was posted on the bulletin board in Bill's room showing the dates the toxin and the stem cells were delivered—the nurse wrote *Happy Re-Birthday!* next to the stem cell date. An uplifting idea—a fresh beginning. One vital fact: transfusions are available to replace red blood cells and platelets, but white blood cells can't be replaced by transfusion; we had to wait for the stem cells to take root in the bone marrow and develop into mature white blood cells. The blood cell calendar records the daily blood counts (white blood cells, red blood cells, and platelets). The normal white blood cell count is about 5,000. The calendar showed Bill's count dropping daily until one day the nurse recorded *less than 0.1*—so low it was unmeasurable. Bill was very weak, unable to eat or drink, and slept nearly all the time. At last, after twelve days, the blood count ticked upward ever so slightly, and Bill was doing better, more alert and responsive. We were elated for a day or two as it appeared the worst was behind us. But this was the calm before the storm. Bill had developed a cough and the chest CT scan was suspicious for pneumonia. After this fleeting improvement, Bill's condition took a turn for the worse.

Driving home from the hospital, I learned my daughter-in-law was in labor; a new grandson quickly arrived. One moment I was consumed by the turn in Bill's symptoms, and the next moment, I was staring at this photo of a new life and the joy of proud new parents. My sister said, *It's like feeling every human emotion in one day.* I'd hoped to travel for a visit when the baby arrived, but when I reached the Transplant Unit the next morning, the oncologist approached in the hall to prepare me before I entered the room. *He looks rough,* he said.

It was a suddenly perilous time. Bill was short of breath, his heart racing, his condition worsening hour by hour. The cause of the pneumonia—the type of infection—was unknown. The white blood cell counts were still very low, so a broad range of antibiotics were employed with no signs of improvement. Among the flurry of diagnostic tests performed, a young oncologist-in-training sent a new test for an unlikely cause, Legionnaires' disease. And this was positive. The antibiotics were adjusted for more specificity as Bill's condition turned critical and he was transferred to the intensive care unit. Imaging showed the lungs being overtaken by infection. Bill needed more and more respiratory support, and even so, he was struggling for air. *The prognosis is poor. There's just a slim chance the antibiotics plus the weak immune system will overcome the spreading infection.* More and more doctors arrived, clustering outside our room and speaking in low voices as we do when things are grave. My own heart jumped each time Bill's heart began to race, I gasped as he strained to take each breath, and I ached to see a glimmer of response when we spoke to him. Emotional numbness settled over me as I focused on each medical detail and did what I believed he would want at each step.

The bacteria causing Legionnaires' disease is found in water systems, so the use of all water in the hospital was abruptly stopped, and cartons and cartons of bottled water were distributed on every floor. The water systems were tested, but the source was never found.

And then, exceeding all expectations, Bill began to improve. Slowly, the infection receded and the whole process went in reverse. He was transferred to an intermediate care unit—so very weak and frail. After a month of hospitalization, he was still very weak but ready to leave. The oncologist nixed transfer to rehabilitation due to risk of infection. We returned home and sat on the couch staring at each other, struggling to absorb what had happened, and almost happened.

CHAPTER 3

•

We Are Dying

RECUPERATION FROM THE bone marrow transplant and the nearly
fatal bout with Legionnaires' disease was slow and arduous. Bill returned home painfully thin, malnourished, incredibly weak, his mus-
cles shriveled, his legs unrecognizably swollen. Week by week he
climbed back to health. He was not as robust as before, but we recognized steady progress.

....

BILL'S JOURNAL

It has been so long since I've written—so many serious things have
come and gone. The BMT—the transplant was a success but the
experience was very difficult—nausea, complete loss of appetite—
I think I didn't eat for three weeks. I developed severe pneumonia,
trouble breathing, high fevers, atrial fibrillation, became enceph-
alopathic, so I remember little of the experience. Lisa and family
watching over me—all extremely important to my recovery. After
a lifetime working in hospitals, I got a good view of how all levels
of staff are needed for the patient to feel cared for—hospital staff
was excellent.

....

Bill was now earmarked as high risk. The plan had been to aggressively follow up with a second bone marrow transplant, but it was clear he was unlikely to survive it. Bill remained at risk for infection for months after the transplant, and we took few chances. Visits with family and friends were by phone and Skype. When we began getting out, it was daunting to see how weak he was. Still, there was progress, and we gradually began to plan again: back-to-back medical conferences in Ireland and Norway were an opportunity for Bill to plan a travel adventure. We also planned to rent a house in Santa Fe where our children and grandchildren would join us.

Bill had survived a close shave with disaster, but our intuition from decades of practicing medicine told us the failed chemotherapy and complicated transplant were poor prognostic signs. By and large, I took the lead from Bill: he showed no willingness to discuss his prognosis or to ponder the future beyond doing our best to get back to our life.

Bill was more about process; I'm more about goal setting. I admired this about Bill and try to emulate it: how he lived in the moment, how he lived with grace, accepting the rhythms of life, its peaks and its valleys. The more I explore his qualities, the more I respect his nuance and subtlety. He was the master of "the grand gesture," delighting everyone with the unexpected, from a bottle of champagne to tickets to Bunraku puppetry in Japan. But to know him was also to recognize the meaning of the small gesture, the subtlety of what he chose to say and when he chose to say it. Even as his health declined, even as he confronted the gravity of illness and pain, even as he lay dying, this was his essence. Less was more.

Through it all, I respected the primacy of Bill's needs. It may be my medical training or my natural inclination to be patient-centered, to respond to individual patient preferences. And it also reflects how we lived our lives: a reciprocal dynamic where the comfort and happiness of the other trumps our own. I scrutinized his behavior—his gestures, his choice of words, his facial expression—for signs of what he needed. There were many things I wanted to say and so many thoughts I wanted to hear. I occasionally dipped my toe in the water to gauge the temperature, and modulated my response to respond to his nuanced signals. And over time, the fine balance of our lives together tilted.

We were uplifted by the day-by-day improvement and began to return to some semblance of normal. On my first day back at work seeing patients, I saw a man in his early 50s with a tremor of one hand. After the history and exam, I explained the diagnosis was Parkinson's disease. The man and his wife held each other closely and cried together. I had made this diagnosis hundreds of times, but this time I thought, *If only that was us.* Even as I felt their sorrow, I wished Bill and I could be in their shoes.

Our unspoken fears were confirmed on a follow-up visit soon after the stem cell transplant. The oncologist explained the lab tests showed an early trend of myeloma cells coming back. Bill was *technically still in remission but . . .* Bill handled this bad news with his usual grace: a brief, soulful acknowledgement, then a deft use of silence. He changed the subject, describing our plans to travel to Europe in the coming weeks. The oncologist questioned the wisdom of our plans, describing travel disasters of other patients, and Bill countered with humor. The oncologist appeared uneasy, as he looked for a sign that we understood what we were facing. *We'll go and we'll just hope for the best,* I said. That seemed to settle him. *Yes, that's right—you will hope for the best.*

The June trip to Ireland and Norway marked the high point of the entire period from diagnosis to Bill's demise. Bill said that from the time of his diagnosis, he never felt normal and "good" again. Nonetheless, this trip was a period of relative well-being where we experienced the familiar joys of travel together. Bill was an extraordinary traveler, quickly getting his bearings in a new city. He had sharp instincts for the places to visit and the food to order—especially the local beer and ale—to make a new destination come alive. We boarded a Hurtigruten ship traveling the Norwegian coast from Bergen to Kirkenes in the far north, just miles from the Russian border. Days of endless sun passed so slowly you could hear yourself think. Each day the ship's intercom announced the main event: waving to the passengers on the sister ship as it passed by traveling in the opposite direction. We glided by narrow fjords and ate *klippfisk*, the dried salted cod that draped over

A-frame racks along the craggy coast. We celebrated our first passage above the Arctic Circle by observing a dubious tradition where the ship's captain poured ice down our backs, to the great amusement of our fellow passengers. And I don't recall a single time we spoke of all things medical—either from our past, present, or future.

....

BILL'S JOURNAL

Time passes so quickly—back from Ireland and Norway—did
well except near the end of the trip in Oslo, I began to have
left leg pain—very reminiscent of the earlier problem with the
right leg—troublesome thoughts.

....

Later that summer, we rented a house in Santa Fe where we were joined by children and grandchildren, and returned to the colorful Indian Market. But as we browsed the stalls at the farmers' market and hiked the trails at Tent Rocks National Monument it was apparent the scales were tipping, as Bill's energy and vigor faded day by day. With the first signs of autumn, we again sat side by side in the synagogue in observance of the Yom Kippur holiday. As we heard the familiar prayer, *who shall live and who shall die*, I turned to Bill: *We're blessed that you recovered after being so ill during this past year.* And he began to cry—the first and the last time I saw him cry.

Two weeks later Bill was feeling unusually well, so we planned a special dinner date to celebrate our wedding anniversary. We toasted with vodka martinis and lost ourselves in chatter over sizzling steaks. And then suddenly, as we sipped coffee, Bill turned pale and ashen. We made it home filled with apprehension as we turned in for the night. Shortly after, we awakened to discover Bill was bleeding internally and I called 911. We surmised he had developed an ulcer, and hemorrhage wasn't surprising since his platelet count (responsible for blood clotting) remained so low. I waited outside the gastrointestinal endoscopy suite, anticipating that report. But instead the gastroenterologist described shocking news: Bill's stomach was filled with bleeding metastatic tumors. Bill was still sedated as I accompanied the stretcher

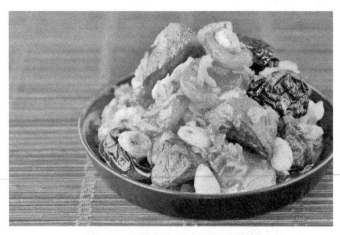

LAMB AND DRIED APRICOT TAGINE
The Jewish New Year, September 2012
Easy to prepare—the results delightful—saffron-scented and
surprisingly spicy with a lingering taste. Lamb is soft & succulent.
Bill & Lisa

back to the ICU. The thought of telling Bill the news when he awoke
from anesthesia was searing. Neither of us were aware that myeloma
cells could cause tumors outside the bone marrow. The oncologist
explained how very rare this is and how it signaled an unusually
aggressive cancer. He described how the myeloma cells had learned
a nasty trick—to grow outside the bone marrow, leaving destruction
in their path. We thought we had longer, but as we listened we knew:
this was the beginning of the end.

The pace of problems and treatments became a blur as blood and
platelet transfusions were needed with increasing frequency—two
times a week, three times a week, then nearly every day. Radiation
therapy was started to shrink the stomach and intestinal tumors. Pink
lines were inked over Bill's body to mark the radiation fields, and I
shuddered to watch him disappear behind the thick iron door that
slowly closed before each radiation treatment.

A large bell is mounted on the wall of radiation oncology; it's rung
by patients to mark the completion of their course of radiation, with
staff and family gathered round. But when the nurses encouraged Bill

to ring the bell, he firmly refused. I didn't understand why. He later explained he recalled our colleague with multiple myeloma ringing that bell—and dying soon after.

THANKSGIVING WAS APPROACHING. There would be no house in the Hudson River Valley this year; instead, all the children and grandchildren joined us in our home in Baltimore. But so many transfusions and treatments were needed; we were spending long days in the hospital. Late Wednesday, the day before Thanksgiving, as Bill eased himself into the car to go home, his weakened collarbone snapped, and he was suddenly in unbearable pain. Instead of driving home to join our waiting family, we were on our way to the emergency room. The following day, heavily medicated, Bill was discharged to return home for the Thanksgiving holiday. The children and grandchildren gathered to greet him in the driveway as we pulled up to our home. They had pulled together to prepare a wonderful dinner . . . but a dinner he couldn't enjoy. As we gathered around the table, each of us recited what we were thankful for this year. And Bill slowly said, *That I am here.*

The next day when we returned to the hospital for blood transfusions, the oncologist was waiting to speak to us. It was time for a decision: hospice care or one final hospitalization for chemotherapy. Bill leaned toward hospice, then reluctantly agreed to again be hospitalized for treatment. Family and friends helped us through this time of little hope, where the goal of preserving the quality of our days became more and more elusive. Bill began to sleep more and more, and I wasn't certain if this was sleep or a gradual withdrawal from everything, including me.

The day came for the oncologist to report the results of this final course of chemotherapy—*there was no response at all.* It was time to discuss arrangements for hospice care. As I sat close to his hospital bed, words cannot capture the desolation of these moments. Even so, I never thought that Bill would ask me to end his life. He described where I would find the morphine at home, that I could bring it back with me. *I cannot do this. I love you.* In those dire moments, I could no longer make sense of what love asks of us. But I couldn't do this for him—and Bill honored that.

Returning home assumed great importance. In the quiet of our home we were surrounded by objects that recapitulated moments of our life together: cherished books, collections, and handicrafts. It never failed to ease Bill's mind to return home, but now, as he needed more care, he insisted it was no longer possible. Seized by resolve, I made all manner of arrangements and lists of symptoms, medications, equipment, and treatments. I would continue to bring Bill to the hospital for transfusions—albeit with reduced frequency—since even short-term survival depended upon it.

The day we returned home, Bill sat in his favorite spot on the couch. As pale and weak as he was, he relaxed and smiled in the quiet and comfort of our home. But there wasn't going to be any respite from the relentless invasion and decline. Sorrow seeped into our home and smothered our hope for a period of quality of life before death. There were a few shining moments during these days of desolation:

The ethical will: During Bill's final hospital stay, our rabbi taught us about an ethical will—the values that are handed down from one generation to another. Our children gathered around the hospital bed and brainstormed what Bill taught us—things that would always stay with us, both small and large. As ideas sprung to mind, we were caught up in the moment. We called them out one by one, bringing smiles to our faces, laughter to our ears, and joy to our hearts. *Be generous—leave big tips. The best food is what you prepare at home. Eat strong, smelly cheese. Be forgiving to yourself and others. Don't take yourself too seriously. Stand by your principles. Express your opinions. Make the "grand gesture." Take public transportation in far-away places. Pause to add meaning to life—with a stiff drink at the end of the day or by lighting Shabbat candles. Be bold . . . Take risks . . . Try new adventures . . .* And as we spoke, Bill lit up in the joy of the moment. He experienced a transfusion of life as he glimpsed his legacy. Indeed, it was what we'd all been searching for: to acknowledge his final days with love and to show in a hundred ways, large and small, how he would live on.

A tribute from our colleagues: Our colleagues planned a tribute to Bill by naming the University of Maryland Neurology Hospital Service in his honor. A ceremony was planned on the campus to present a plaque to Bill in a few weeks, but I sensed we needed to proceed immediately. Two days later and just a week before he died, one hundred people arrived at our home to honor Bill. As the time of the event arrived, Bill was very weak and withdrawn. I asked if he could manage this and he slowly shook his head *no*. But as the guests arrived and came over to speak to him one by one, he was energized and restored right before our eyes. After several speakers extolled his accomplishments, he was invited to speak. People say that before death, remarkable moments of rejuvenation occur—and this was Bill's moment. He spoke off the cuff, dissolving the melancholy in the room, reminiscing about special moments with colleagues, making everyone comfortable . . . *Aren't you supposed to wait until someone's gone to do this*? He was back. It was transcendent.

In the final days, we were challenged again and again to make the time meaningful, to show our love, to help him find peace. To nourish his body and soul, Bill's daughters whipped up an appetizing array of shakes and smoothies. And it calmed me to watch Bill's daughter sit by his bedside and begin to read *Anna Karenina* to him. A smile played on Bill's lips as he listened and imagined hearing the last of the eight hundred pages.

And I sat by him, telling him stories of our life together: the romance, the excitement, the joy. I watched his face relax and reflect as I described our experiences, with anecdotes that captured who he was and who we were together.

The decline over the final days was so rapid that every day brought new problems—Bill was weaker and weaker, speaking less and less, sleeping more and more, refusing food or drink. As I strained to lay him back in bed, the gravity of our situation struck me anew. My thoughts escaped in a wail of sorrow: *What am I going to do?* Seized by an unnatural power, Bill abruptly sat up. With an expression of ferocity, his eyes bore into mine and he jabbed his finger in my face. He spoke in the loud, strident voice that was long gone . . . *Now, that is the right question*. Stunned, I froze in my spot as he lay down, exhausted.

On December 27, 2012, we had an appointment to go to the hospital for transfusions. I didn't know what to do. Bill was so ill and dazed. How would I transport him? I struggled to confront where we had arrived—*finality*. Could I abandon hope—even the hope for just a few more days? I yearned to discuss this with Bill, to face this with him, to do what he wanted. Suppressing hopelessness one last time, I dressed him and transferred him into the car and the hospital with help from doormen on both ends. When we arrived in the cancer center, the nurses looked horrified. Bill's last lab results were so bad that someone was supposed to call us . . . to tell us not to come in . . . that it was hopeless. But no one called.

We were placed in a cubicle with the curtain closed around us— like we needed to be isolated from everyone . . . from the staff, from the patients.

A nurse came to tell us this news: *There won't be any more transfusions.*

As ill as he was, he understood. Bill was saying very little, but now he said, *It's time to go home.*

The trip home was unspeakable.

I strained to think clearly—to do the right thing.

The bottom was falling out from under us. That night, Bill was terribly agitated, continually asking to move from place to place—no sleep at all.

The next morning, I sat at our kitchen table, staring and struggling to comprehend. I called our rabbi and choked on the words: *I need help. I don't know what to do. I think I need to plan a funeral.*

The rabbi's response: *I'm coming over.*

We sat at the kitchen table, where the rabbi described in simple language what needed to be done. He asked if he could go into the bedroom to pray with Bill. *Of course, but I don't know if Bill is able to participate.* We sat Bill on the side of the bed, supported between the two of us. The rabbi explained the Viddui, a prayer recited when death is imminent. The Viddui is a confessional, acknowledging the imperfections of the dying and seeking a final reconciliation with God. When the rabbi began to recite the traditional prayer—the Shema, *Hear O Israel, the Lord is our God, the Lord is One*—Bill mouthed every word.

The two miracles of Bill's final days were the tribute from our colleagues the week before he died, and the time with the rabbi on Bill's final day, December 28. Weeks later I sent a note to the rabbi: *I'm certain you've done many mitzvot* (good deeds) *in your life, but you'll never do anything that surpasses the importance of those moments with Bill.*

> For three whole days, during which time did not exist for him, he struggled in that black sack into which he was being thrust by an invisible, resistless force . . . He felt that his agony was due to his being thrust into that black hole and still more to his not being able to get right into it. He was hindered from getting into it by his conviction that his life had been a good one. That very justification of his life held him fast and prevented his moving forward, and it caused him most torment of all. Suddenly some force struck him in the chest and side, making it still harder to breathe, and he fell through the hole and there at the bottom was a light.
>
> —LEO TOLSTOY, *The Death of Ivan Ilyich*

Can we be prepared for the finality of death? In the dead of night, Bill again became fitful and agitated, struggling to get out of bed. I ripped opened the "comfort pack" that hospice left in our refrigerator, straining to focus on the different medicine bottles fitted with glass droppers. *Which drugs and which dosages would bring comfort?* But the restlessness continued. Taking long heavy breaths, he murmured and motioned his need to move around our room. We moved back and forth from the hospital bed to our bed. And I went back and forth to the comfort pack, reading the instructions time and time again to find the right formula. Frantic and sleepless, I struggled to decipher what was happening—what I could do to bring him peace. As he lay beside me in bed, I held him and comforted him to no avail . . . and then he said a single clear sentence, *I'm trapped in a cage.* And as those cryptic words turned over and over in my mind, he was gone.

> The timing of death, like the ending of a story, gives a changed meaning to what preceded it.
>
> —MARY CATHERINE BATESON

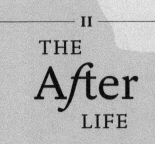

II

THE
After
LIFE

GRIEF AND LOSS

CHAPTER 4

◆

The Altered Life

I peer out the window on a bus and see the approaching destination—an unfamiliar skyline. When we arrive, the bus driver walks down the aisle to my seat—he's annoyed. He says my behavior is unacceptable, that I've been cursing and swearing loudly. I'm unaware of any of this—*I might have been thinking these things, but not saying them out loud.* The driver glares at me and blocks me from getting off the bus. Suddenly Bill walks down the aisle and is standing right in front of me. He looks wonderful—brimming with health. He's wearing his blue sport jacket, white shirt, and burgundy tie with colored dots. He looks at me lovingly and smiles, filling me with joy. I cry out to the driver, *Do you see him?* And then, Bill is gone.

I now understand what's happening: I think I'm behaving normally but this isn't the reality. I'm behaving strangely, saying bizarre things, seeing Bill when he's not there.

Others see something's wrong with me.

MY NEED TO BRING BILL HOME from the hospital after that final round of chemotherapy was unequivocal. And though I understood Bill was dying, I didn't think through or envision how things would end—that after his death, strangers would arrive in our home to take him away. They arrived in the dead of night and they were all business. They asked me if I wanted to stay or leave our bedroom while they did their job. Dazed, I wondered *Why would I leave him now?* And then they put him in a stiff opaque bag and pulled the long zipper closed. As the zipper covered his face, I lurched forward in horror: *DON'T DO THAT.* They'd seen this before—this disruption. *You'll need to leave the room now . . .* I watched them roll the stretcher out the door of our home and into the van, and as the rear lights receded in the darkness, Bill's daughters said in small voices, *Goodbye, Daddy.*

We were sitting in stunned silence when there was another knock on the door in the middle of the night. As a woman brushed past me, she identified herself as a hospice worker. She walked straight to the kitchen refrigerator, removed the comfort pack, and threw its contents down the toilet. And as the toilet flushed behind her, she silently walked out the door. *They fear I'm going to use that,* I thought, recalling the overflowing cabinet of Bill's drugs in the next room.

The funeral was scheduled for Sunday, December 30. On the last day of Bill's life, after the rabbi led us in prayer, Bill had suddenly gripped my arm and strained to say, *A cemetery.* We didn't have gravesites. We'd never discussed this. His face, his voice, was so plaintive, so troubled. Even now, he was taking care of things. I steadied my voice to sound assured. *I know—I'll take care of everything.* You've always made me feel protected, now it's my turn to make you feel safe.

As the sun rose on that first day without Bill, we had a full day planned: funeral home, cemeteries, grave sites, and time with the rabbi to reminisce. I moved through the weekend's events one by one. The next day: dressing for the funeral, greeting family and friends, listening to eulogies, gathering in the cemetery. My soul shuddered as Bill's casket descended into the frozen earth. I sensed some moral responsibility to maintain decorum, but in the recesses of my mind, I wasn't part of the funeral procession. I was with Bill, not with the mourners. And I was talking to Bill when I recited my eulogy:

I am a lucky woman.

I will always be a lucky woman for having this man in my life and I am a different person for having known him.

Bill,

I will remember.

I will guide others, speak my conscience, and show your kindness and generosity.

I will savor the aching beauty of the crescent moon in the night sky and pause to witness the patterns of the autumn foliage and the changing of the tides.

When I travel far and wide, I will sample the regional food, use the subway, and find those restaurants that only the locals know about. I will pray in the local synagogue, study the local crafts, and check out the farmers' market.

And I will continue to follow in your footsteps, searching for opportunities for all those great new adventures and opportunities for new knowledge—

And I will be looking for you.

I only remember one thing said to me that day by the many colleagues, friends, and family. It was said by one person in hundreds; I'd never seen her before and don't know who she is. *My husband died a year and half ago. I know how you feel today. I can tell you—it will take time, but one day you'll begin to feel better.*

As I changed into comfortable clothes after the funeral, I found an old note from Bill. The sticky note, one of many that Bill tucked into bags of snacks he loved to surprise me with, had strangely found its way into the purse I carried that day. I'd saved this note from a day many years earlier when I traveled to be with my son during illness. Surely more than coincidence, and precisely what Bill wanted to tell me on the day of his funeral.

I miss you. Things will go well! I love you.

Over the next days, the hollowness of our home was masked by the voices of friends and family, the laughter of children, and the reflection of prayer. Sitting in a circle each evening, we poured glasses of the spirits that Bill savored, toasting him and reminiscing—telling

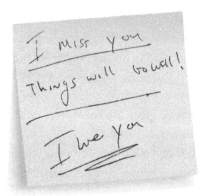

A note from
Bill to Lisa

our stories. But there was no relief from *the invisible blanket between the world and me*, described by C. S. Lewis in *A Grief Observed*. With effort, conversation proceeded, but I was often compelled to tell the story of Bill's last hours over and over. Telling and retelling, describing and redescribing—more to myself than to others. Working to absorb, grasp, take in what happened. Then moments later, I was reflexively looking for Bill in the crowd or making a mental note to tell him about this or that. At other times, I'd be chatting in the most ordinary way—but before long an uneasy sense that something was out of place would wash over me—and then, *I'd remember.* Not wanting to be alone . . . not wanting to be with others . . . *not wanting to be.*

We're talking about the tearing apart of human relationships, where lives are merged and death is eternal separation; where the survivor is left as a fragment, less than whole. This stark reality can be missed in the well-meaning efforts to comfort the dying, to memorialize the dead, and to support the bereaved. As survivors, *we aren't recovering from loss—we are lost.* We wake up to a world we don't recognize, where entrenched habits and behaviors are obsolete.

I drove my son, the final departing guest, to the airport. Later in the week, I planned to travel to spend more time with family. Bill and I had no family in Baltimore; we were simply a complete unit—the two of us. As I pulled away from the airport, the road spread out before me like the future, aimless and alien. The routines and habits of a lifetime were upended; I was purposeless, unmoored. The last thing I recall was straining to focus on what I should do that day, that week, that month, that year . . . and then, I became aware I was in the car, driving somewhere I didn't recognize. I'd lost track of time and place and couldn't get my bearings; I felt a rising sense of anxiety as my mind froze and basic problem-solving was out of reach. I took the next exit off the highway and pulled over to gather my thoughts. The GPS led me home. I struggled to perceive what was happening; my behavior was utterly foreign and I was dazed by my lack of control, my incoherence.

Two days later, I packed to visit my children. But when the time came to leave for the airport, I sat next to my suitcase, unable to find the will to walk out the door. This made no sense—this irrational disconnect between my decisions and my behavior. I forced myself to walk to the door and froze again with my hand on the doorknob. *I couldn't leave.* Minutes went by—*what was happening?* And then on an impulse, I called out loudly, *Bill, we're leaving. We're going to visit the children.* And only then, I walked out, locking the door behind me.

And with that, the altered life began: waking up each day in an unfamiliar world where all rules are scrambled. Where you can no more connect with yourself than with those around you. Where the default is a sense of alienation, not fitting in the world. Where a simple chat involves navigating land mines, and life's routine stories are fraught with emotion. Each utterance preceded by split-second analyses—*Can I say this sentence without breaking down? Will the listener be too distressed to hear this?* Perpetually self-conscious, since all stories circle back to life with Bill—or without him. I circumvented each thought and phrase that came to mind, pausing and faltering. I experimented with using *I* instead of *we* to avoid conjuring up emotions; the result was a strained stammer—*our home . . . well, my home, when we . . . when I traveled.* It was a long time before I told a simple story from the past with a firm voice. I was unable to refer to Bill as if he was gone. With time, I was less spontaneous, more quiet in social situations, living more and more inside my head.

It's a testament to the human capacity for attachment. We say our partners make us *complete*, failing to notice the vulnerability of one day finding ourselves *incomplete*.

I think I am beginning to understand why grief feels
like suspense. It comes from the frustration of so
many impulses that had become habitual. Thought
after thought, feeling after feeling, action after action,
had H. for their object. Now their target is gone. I keep
on through habit fitting an arrow to the string, then
I remember and have to lay the bow down. So many
roads lead thought to H. . . . So many roads once;
now so many *culs de sac.*
                                    —C. S. Lewis, *A Grief Observed*

I can't be the same person without Bill in this world loving me.

I'm searching for healing and restoration, but *I'm diminished and damaged by this loss.* I want to honor Bill and to honor what he wanted—to learn from this experience and be a better person for it. But I'm haunted by watching Bill's body decline while he remained who he was. Now I live in the reverse: the person damaged; the vessel intact. I miss the woman I was with Bill. I mourn the loss of that identity—that woman died with him.

When we travel to far-off, exotic places, impressions linger. And living with death and dying was like that: like living in a place so foreign that the effects endured, and I continue to live part of life on this other side. I continue to live with Bill, in an inner world where, from moment to moment, I'm conscious of his response to the day's events, to how my life unfolds. He continues to guide me. I was his muse; now, he is mine.

Life has diminished value. I make a dispassionate appraisal of the purpose of starting a new day. Then I put one foot in front of the other in the hope that tomorrow will be better. Daytime hours are purposeful; determination surfaces. But in the middle of the night, life is meaningless, and I wonder why I go on. The line between optimism and hopelessness is thin. I imagine how Bill would handle this situation—where I'm gone and he's facing life without me. And our separation is so wrenching, the desolation so profound, that if given the choice, I'd choose to switch places with Bill, creating an alternate scenario where he confronts this emptiness and I find peace.

Rituals of grief begin reflexively, without conscious thought: wearing Bill's watch and his clothes, sitting in his chair at our kitchen table or his spot on the couch, pouring his evening glass of scotch, ordering more books than will ever be read. Filling his void by mirroring his behavior. I hunger for information about him. One day, *The Rubáiyát of Omar Khayyám* catches my eye on our library shelf; I open it to find Bill's handwritten note to me tucked in its pages.

> *LXXIII*
>
> *Ah, Love! Could thou and I with Fate conspire*
> *To grasp this sorry Scheme of Things entire,*
> *Would not we shatter it to bits—and then*
> *Re-mould it nearer to the Heart's Desire!*

I feel most alive in these moments, sustaining our bond. Our home is a private sanctuary—the place where we're alone. At times, I'm unsettled by the oddness of my behavior. I follow instinct doing things that bring comfort, but I recognize these rituals may appear peculiar to others. These rituals are likely to be evolutionary and hard-wired. When a herd of elephants encounters an elephant carcass, they stop to tenderly run their trunks across the dry bones. Certain possessions and events assume special, even mystical meaning. Like when I found Bill's note in my purse after his funeral. Or when I returned to an Inuit art gallery Bill loved, to find the sculpture that was meant to come home with me—*The Grieving Woman*.

Instinctively, I follow rituals that soothe me but also blur the boundaries between Bill and me,

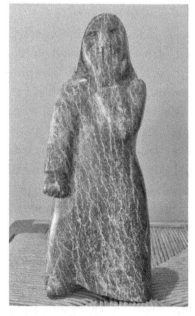

Oviloo Tunnillie, *The Grieving Woman.*

being nourished by old memories instead of creating new ones. The psychologists Amos Tversky and Daniel Kahneman describe common patterns of human irrationality using the term *heuristics* to explain how our minds can fool us. Our predispositions and biases connect the dots to create narratives, to see cause and effect where it may not exist. Our natural inclination is to make a story from events around us, overlooking information that isn't available. The vulnerability of grief is fertile soil for these narratives. *Synchronicity* describes how events during times of grieving may assume special meaning. Dreams and synchronistic events suggest an enduring life energy beyond rational understanding. We suspend disbelief to derive comfort from the unknowable. Our tendency to create these rituals and narratives is sustaining in the setting of loss.

Each day I awaken to find myself *through the looking glass*— a quiet observer of the surreality of this new life. The day starts; I glimpse Bill's eyeglasses next to our bed and his razor by the sink and I sit down for breakfast across from his empty chair. Work is a scaffold to build each day around, but colleagues and staff are also grieving for Bill. I feel like a specter in the office, the sight of me eliciting pained expressions and sorrow.

A month after Bill's death, I resume travel to meetings. Using the airport kiosk, the flight confirmation number retrieves boarding passes *for both Bill and me*—I forgot that months before we had planned to travel together. I struggle to explain what happened to the agent. She asks for Bill's death certificate in the same breath she requests my baggage information, as a matter of course. At moments like this, my mind and body move in different directions—time slows, my mind freezes, and voice and body are on automatic pilot. An altered state where I strain to perform the most ordinary of tasks.

Bill managed our finances. He'd just begun to orient me to what was what when things spun out of control. But even if I was on top of things, financial chaos was inevitable. In these early days, social security payments are deposited one day then clawed back, medical and funeral expenses mount while checks in the mail can't be cashed, my health insurance policy is cancelled since Bill was the primary beneficiary on our family policy. My hands are tied at every step. Calls to manage our accounts yield an officious voice: *You need to put Mr. Weiner on the phone . . . Oh, in that case, bring his death certificate to our office.* But the real problem isn't the bureaucracy, it is the anguish of making call after call to notify AT&T, Visa, American Express that Bill no longer exists. As I toss Bill's ID and credit cards in the trash, I have a palpable sense of contributing to a slow death.

Following loss, how should we behave . . . what is normal? Simple daily interactions are disorienting: responding to personal condolences, being sensitive to the grief of others, awkward transitions to normal conversation. How to find the right balance between expressing too much and too little?

My Condolences

Hundreds of condolences—cards, e-mail messages, thoughtful remarks—all *unwelcome*. Unopened cards pile up on the dining room table. But I can't avoid the chance meeting—without warning, plunged into the pool of grief, turned inside-out. In the most ordinary moment of the day, I'm blessedly distracted—but the sight of me sparks pangs of loss in others. These are mind-numbing, awkward moments. Then there are moments where others share personal memories when we bump into each other on the sidewalk or wait for an elevator. These stories reanimate Bill, piercing my armor.

Condolences—what is their purpose . . . who do they serve? I'm moved when I sense the grief of others, but I envy how they touch down in my world and return to theirs. Condolences don't begin to fill a canyon of loss. I want to extend condolences, not receive them. Expressing condolences eases loss, feels virtuous. No such relief for the recipient. Each message cleaves my union with Bill, tearing apart what I hold on to, bit by bit. There are two sides to each condolence—one side reignites the grief, the other beckons to turn away from the dead and join the living.

Following traumatic loss, we search for comfort; interpersonal and societal expectations shouldn't compound the difficulties. But personal grief may clash with cultural norms and customs. We may feel compelled to conform to social norms for fear of further losses—loss of social support or career opportunities. We may sense the impatience of others with the length of our grieving process. It's difficult to make sound decisions about the right time to return to the workplace, and when we return, coworkers may be concerned about our capacity to manage job responsibilities. We wonder whether we should take on new challenges to engage our minds or defer opportunities. Does loss and grief make us appear weak and vulnerable? Should we mask our grief to avoid alarming family, friends, and colleagues?

CONTACT WITH FRIENDS and family increases soon after a death due to customs and ceremonies. Family members tend to focus on the personal needs of the bereaved, while friends tend to focus on shared activities. A study compared the effects of *friendship* and *kinship* on adjustment following loss of a partner. The researchers predicted that friends would have greater influence on emotional outcomes of grief and depression, and family would have greater influence on coping, self-esteem, and managing grief. Although family was important for both outcomes, the study showed that friendship was a stronger predictor of both, possibly related to more enduring access to friends than family.

> There was this one friend who came to me, after asking permission to do so, every afternoon about four o'clock, sat me down in a chair in the living room, took off my shoes and socks and massaged my feet. He hardly ever said anything. He was a Quaker elder. And yet out of his intuitive sense, he from time to time would say a very brief word like, "I can feel your struggle today," or farther down the road, "I feel that you're a little stronger at this moment, and I'm glad for that." But beyond that, he would say hardly anything. He would give no advice. Somehow he found the one place in my body, namely the soles of my feet, where I could experience some

sort of connection to another human being. And the act of massaging just, you know, in a way that I really don't have words for, kept me connected with the human race.

—KRISTA TIPPETT, *Becoming Wise:*
An Inquiry into the Mystery and Art of Living

Grief is isolating, even though loss is a natural part of life and grief is normal adaptation. Our culture values close friendships and intimate partnerships—grief is simply their echo. But our perception of isolation may be out of proportion to reality; an international study of public expectations of grief showed most people are willing to be with people during grief, regardless of how much time passed since the loss.

Returning to work, returning to my customary roles as neurologist, educator, and researcher, was sustenance to me. As a neurologist, the rigor of making a diagnosis, managing complex symptoms, and living in someone else's shoes for a time was the respite and therapy I needed. As an educator, I found relief in demonstrating key features of the patient's exam and responding to questions from medical

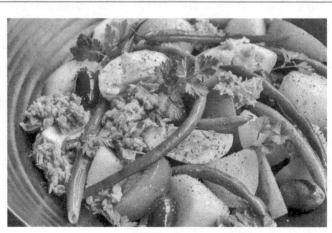

SALADE NIÇOISE
April 2013
Made vinaigrette too salty. Try again.
Just me

students and residents. As a researcher, I lost myself in asking big questions and designing studies to answer them. In performing these roles, I escaped the ever-present emotional quicksand. And remarkably, this sustained itself even though Bill's presence loomed as large in my work as it did in our personal life. There were times when the intersection of our personal and business lives was tricky. With Bill gone, many of his long-time patients began to see me for their care, and they were experiencing their own loss of a trusted physician. Some, but not all, understood we were married. Either way, routine patient care included commiseration about mutual losses. And each time I saw one of his patients, I noted the date Bill wrote his last note about them, reliving where we were in his disease course, imagining how he'd felt that day.

One day I listened to the history of a new patient, an 80-year-old woman who described losing her husband when she was in her 50s. She told me this story: When her husband lay dying, her friend said to her, *Anna, you have to save yourself.* As I listened to her, it seemed as if she had been sent to me to give me this message. I told her I lost my husband a few months before. She looked into my eyes and said, *Dr. Shulman, you have to save yourself. My husband is my heritage. I used what I learned from him to create a new life. Now you must do the same.*

Grief is generally perceived as deep sorrow, but sorrow only captures the emotional impact, not the disorientation and loss of self. *Is it possible that the trauma and disorientation of loss is based in science—not only the biology of sorrow but also a biology of intimacy?* We can envision biologic changes resulting from strong mutualistic relationships, changes resulting from intimate physical and emotional bonding. *Is loss a physiologic process of withdrawal from strong emotional and physical bonds?* These lines of thought help us make sense of the trauma of losing those closest to us—so close that in their absence, we lose ourselves.

A premise of this book is that healing is enhanced by scientific perspectives that help us understand the mechanisms of emotional trauma. We'll continue further down this path to understand what's happening to our mind, brain, and body and to shed light on *the neurology of grief.*

CHAPTER 5

•

The Neurology of Grief

ONE EVENING, I GATHERED INGREDIENTS to prepare a recipe that was one of our favorites: caramelized endive, apples, and grapes served with crusty bread and blue cheese. Standing at the kitchen counter, I opened the cookbook, Dorie Greenspan's *Around My French Table*, to the recipe and found Bill's familiar scribble at the top of the page.

Then time passed with no conscious awareness . . .

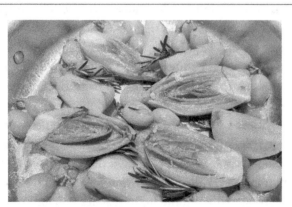

CARAMELIZED ENDIVE, APPLES, AND GRAPES
August 9, 2011
Our first "as if" dinner after our return from Maine—
the menu was the same and it was as delicious as ever.
Bill & Lisa

- While awake, I sometimes feel like I'm in a dream.
- I feel emotionally numb.
- I find myself in places without knowing how I got there.
- Time goes by without my awareness.
- I have trouble focusing or concentrating.
- I feel detached or estranged from people.
- I feel like I'm on automatic pilot.
- I feel like an observer of my own life.

Dissociating offers an escape hatch from the thoughts and memories we're not ready to face. Our subconscious mind senses what we can and cannot handle, and even perceives when we're ready to cope with painful information. We all have triggers that activate defense mechanisms. We may be aware of some triggers while being unaware of others. A trigger, such as seeing a certain photo or returning to a special place, may cause a sudden change of mood. We may sense rising anxiety or even panic, and experience a strong urge to get away from the situation. Since we may be unaware of the trigger, our powerful emotional response can be frightening. We also have everyday defense mechanisms that we use regularly to manage the stress of our lives, but these mechanisms typically don't cause emotional disruption.

It's no wonder these coping mechanisms become more elaborate in the face of traumatic loss. Defense mechanisms are vital adaptations. With healing and restoration, people's need for these mechanisms slowly wanes. Strong triggers may continue to elicit these responses, but with time, the manifestations of dissociation will generally become less potent.

From a neurologist's perspective, the experience of grieving is easier to understand. All emotional and psychiatric symptoms have correlates in brain function. What we often experience during grief corresponds to many common neurologic deficits: the fog of *confusion*, the *inattention*, the *visual neglect* (holes in my visual field that block perception of Bill's personal belongings around the house). And then, the *delusions* of *magical thinking* described by Joan Didion, who kept her husband's shoes in the closet in case he returned. We vacillate from the comfort of magical thinking to the uneasy feeling we're not making sense—*that we're going crazy.*

> I realized for the time being I could not trust myself
> to present a coherent face to the world.
> —JOAN DIDION, *The Year of Magical Thinking*

This sense of incoherence arises during emotionally charged situations following traumatic loss. In the following examples, the emotional fog of grief disrupts attention and clarity of thought.

Bill's things: I feel both repelled and compelled to attend to Bill's clothes. The touch of his shirt, a vest or scarf, summons the sense he'll walk in any moment. It's intimate and jarring. To calm a rising emotional storm, I obsessively catalogue the items on spreadsheets. When I hesitate to part with something, it stays in the closet. The room piles high with boxes and garment bags. My insides in a knot, I struggle to narrow my focus on the basic task: donating clothes. I unload the car at Goodwill, and as the first bags are thrown into the large bin, I panic and flee with the overflowing trolley. *I can't leave these things in this impersonal place.* I drive away in a frenzy. When I arrive at our apartment, on an impulse, I give the doorman all of Bill's things. We say nothing about where twenty-two bags of clothes came from. I don't explain and he doesn't ask, but he knows. And that's enough.

The symbolism of gravestones: My voice quivers as I phone the monument store to purchase a headstone for Bill's grave. The salesman asks, *And who is this for?* Several weeks later, the salesman calls to say the headstone arrived: *You may want to inspect it before we deliver it to the cemetery.* The headstone is locked in a small fenced-in area surrounded by others. I stare in disbelief. I pace back and forth around the fence, seized by a powerful impulse to break in and rescue Bill from this pen. Reason and intellect are no match for this mounting sense of urgency.

Grief and the hazards of distraction: Five months after Bill's death, I travel to Sydney, Australia, to give a talk. Upon arrival, I self-consciously walk in Bill's footsteps, stopping at the concierge, asking

Bill's usual questions: *Do you have any suggestions for a nice walk . . . restaurants the locals go to . . . galleries with local crafts?* Armed with a map with circled highlights, I head to the harbor and up into the city, where a street fair beckons. And then . . . I fall. I step off the cobblestone curb and my ankle twists with a sickening crunch. People run to help me. I'm anguished by visions of Bill watching me and feeling helpless. And then I realize: I am helpless. I'm alone halfway around the world and I'm injured. I stand up uncertainly. I walk for a block but my foot swells and no longer fits in the shoe. The hotel concierge finds me limping across the lobby; the X-ray shows a fractured ankle. People say grief increases risk for falls and accidents. That year, I not only fall but also hit a wall with my car . . . twice.

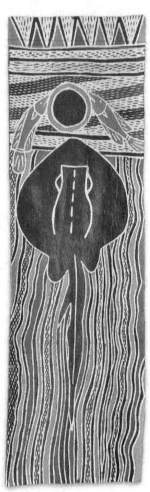

Before leaving Australia, I clomp up to the podium (to talk about disability, no less). Despite my injury, I continue a tradition of bringing a memento home from each destination. My interpretation of the Aboriginal bark painting I select: Bill and I are the fish building our life together, oblivious to the ominous sting ray approaching. *No,* Bill's daughter says reassuringly. *It's two lovely fish guiding the sting ray up the river.*

Grief takes up a lot of bandwidth in the brain. Odd behavior and incoherence are expected consequences of the brain's protective responses following emotional trauma. During these times, my behavior often doesn't make sense to me. The line between feeling in control and feeling lost is very thin. I seesaw from one extreme to another. At both

Aboriginal bark painting
memento from Australia

extremes, I'm deluded. First, I'm back on my feet, then I'm toppled by a wave of despair. After many cycles, it's best to anticipate this pattern, mindful that neither the worst nor the best of times will endure.

Recovery from loss—the experience, symptoms, and duration—is as diverse as the individual circumstances. It's common for people to wonder if what they're experiencing is *normal* or *outside the norm*. Responses to loss lie on a continuum: many people have emotional responses that are limited in severity and duration, and others have more intense responses of longer duration. The following sections describe recovery from significant loss and more sustained forms of emotional trauma.

COMPLICATED GRIEF AND POST-TRAUMATIC STRESS DISORDER

Complicated grief (CG) and post-traumatic stress disorder (PTSD) are usually described as separate, unrelated disorders, with different diagnostic criteria for each listed in psychiatric manuals. However, CG and PTSD are closely linked. They are natural responses to unusually traumatic circumstances. Many symptoms overlap between these disorders, including the experience of emotional numbness and the presence of triggers. Dissociation is common in both CG and PTSD. PTSD flashbacks are described as surges of emotion from an earlier traumatic experience. This echoes the disconnect of feelings from thoughts in response to triggers of dissociation in complicated grief.

Complicated grief—where grief becomes stalled, behaving more like a chronic condition than a brief, limited condition—by definition lasts more than six months. Chronic neurologic disorders like chronic traumatic encephalopathy (CTE) also have overlapping symptoms with traumatic loss. Encephalopathy is a broad neurologic term describing abnormal brain function due to many different causes; it may be reversible, stable, or progressive. CTE is a consequence of concussion, often a sports-related injury, and is a hot topic in the news recently.

The definition of concussion is expanding, encompassing causes that include not only direct physical trauma, like a blow to the head, but also injuries from a blast or jolt. And the list of CTE aftereffects is also expanding, from temporary unconsciousness to feeling dazed or confused. It's not a big step to include *emotional shock*, or severe emotional trauma, in this definition, where changes in brain function (altered mental status, encephalopathy) from psychological trauma result in the confusion and incapacity associated with any of these diagnostic categories—CTE, PTSD, or CG.

Whether physical or emotional, *brain trauma is trauma*. Trauma results in brain injury—changes in brain function—and there are a finite number of ways the brain responds to trauma. The key questions are whether these changes in brain function are reversible and how we can enhance recovery and healing.

> In the diagnostic procedure we are not carving at the
> joints of nature. Diagnostic categories are invented
> and arbitrary; they are a product of committee vote
> and invariably undergo considerable revision with each
> passing decade . . . the chore of making a formal diagnosis
> is more than a simple nuisance. It may, in fact, impede
> our work by obscuring, even negating, the full-bodied,
> multidimensional individual facing us in our office.
> —IRVIN D. YALOM, *Creatures of a Day*

Clinicians create criteria for diagnosis and management, but these criteria have little relevance in our daily lives. All traumatic loss has some features of complicated grief and post-traumatic stress disorder. There is a spectrum or range of symptoms of trauma and grief in everyone experiencing traumatic loss.

RECOVERY AND HEALING

How can we recover and lessen the power traumatic memories have over us? Healing involves transforming traumatic memories into less emotionally charged memories. Since these memories have emotional components that are dissociated from their cognitive counterparts, recovery involves reconnecting the emotional and cognitive components so that painful memories are gradually reintegrated into conscious awareness.

From a neurologic perspective, traumatic memories create their own neural pathways: certain triggers activate brain pathways associated with anxiety and even a *fight or flight* response. Healing results from *neuroplasticity*, or the capacity for remodeling and rewiring neural pathways. This reconnection of emotional and cognitive components of memory can be achieved in many ways, including seeing a counselor, journaling, or simply returning to meaningful life experiences that nurture a sense of confidence and safety.

Importantly, recent studies show that dissociation is not associated with poorer outcomes. Rather, in a study of people with complicated grief, *the presence of dissociation was associated with a better response to psychotherapeutic treatment*. People experiencing dissociation may have the most to gain from therapies that raise awareness and enhance processing of loss. Similarly, studies show the most effective treatments for PTSD involve cognitive-behavioral therapy, in which people are gradually exposed to traumatic memories in an attempt to create new associations and reduce their emotional charge. Dissociation is likely to be an important protective response during grief: an internal gauge or filter that referees when we're ready for painful memories to get through.

PREDICTING OUTCOMES AFTER TRAUMATIC LOSS

For many years, conventional wisdom held that people must deliberately explore and work through emotional trauma. Conversely, avoiding emotions associated with traumatic events was believed to increase and sustain psychiatric symptoms. From this perspective, defense mechanisms like dissociation were viewed as maladaptive, increasing the risk of post-traumatic stress disorder and prolonged grief. More recently, these views have changed; increasingly, experts accept that avoidance plays an important role in helping people adapt to traumatic loss and is a normal part of mourning. Recent studies don't support theories claiming that avoidance (less emotional distress during bereavement) results in worse outcomes. Instead, *studies show that emotional avoidance may support adaptation by providing the means to regulate the amount of emotional stress we're ready to experience over time.*

Avoiding stressors can be accomplished in many ways, from suppressing painful thoughts to seeking out simple distraction. These strategies may be subconscious or conscious, such as discovering that time with certain friends relieves stress while being with others has quite the opposite effect. Dissociation and other defense mechanisms are subconscious ways that people avoid stress. These are key strategies that enable us to continue to function at work and at home. From this perspective, avoiding unpleasant emotions might not be a bad thing.

Grief work is important after loss, but it's also important to honor the readiness and unique pace of the individual. People experiencing more severe grief, including emotional dissociation, are likely to need more time to express thoughts and memories after loss. *But here's the key thing—as useful as avoidance and distraction may be, we can't delay integration, processing, and awareness forever. Finding ways to express feelings, thoughts, and memories is the bedrock of growth and healing.* Each of us has our own "dosing regimen" with the right dose and the right time frame, but we won't heal without means of expression and insight. For me, writing is the best outlet, but there are countless vehicles for expression, from speaking to a trusted listener to creating unique artistic expressions of your emotions by drawing or composing music.

For my part, I see tangible progress: sometimes I'm engaged in this new life and I find renewed strength to talk and reminisce about life with Bill. Then I think, *I'm recovering—look how far I've come.* But then, without notice, a sense of unreality washes over me as I'm struck anew by how life has changed. As C. S. Lewis wrote, *Tonight all the hells of young grief have opened again . . . For in grief nothing 'stays put.' One keeps on emerging from a phase, but it always recurs. Round*

and round. Everything repeats . . . The same leg is cut off time after time.
After many cycles of buoyancy to bleakness, I recognize this familiar
pattern. And at both extremes, I remind myself—*don't overthink this
. . . it will pass.* I give myself permission to have these moments. Bill
was forgiving of himself—I try to be forgiving of myself.

Recovery, healing, restoration take time—and I've come to see
this process as a long journey. As the years pass, the fog recedes and
reveals at first small glimpses, then growing awareness, of who we are,
where we've been, and where we're going—as a new stage of growth
is born from loss.

In this chapter and the chapters to follow, I describe *three principles to heal the mind and brain after loss and to promote insight and
awareness*:

1. *Subconscious–Conscious Integration*
2. *Immersion–Distraction*
3. *Opening the Mind to Possibilities*

Traumatic loss results in blocked access to painful emotions and
memories. This response is protective in the short-term but detrimental to healthy function in the long-term. The first principle,
Subconscious–Conscious Integration, describes the need to gradually
surface painful experiences, restoring them to conscious memory
where they can be reintegrated into our life story. The second principle, *Immersion–Distraction*, describes the strategy to accomplish this
reintegration. This is a purposeful, gradual process of dedicating time
to dwell on traumatic emotions and memories where one recollection
slowly unlocks another. This involves deliberately going down a disturbing path, so equal attention is needed for times of rest and rejuvenation (distraction). Mindful inner work will be elevated by periods
of diversion. The third principle, *Opening the Mind to Possibilities*,
describes the gradual process of turning a corner to rebuild personal
identity and to contemplate new options for the future.

A Pause for Journaling*

Describe times when your defense mechanisms appear and describe the triggers you're aware of—sights, sounds, people, or events that cause you to experience heightened anxiety and agitation. Explore why these events tend to trigger heightened emotions.

*Pauses for journaling encourage you to set aside some time to reflect on how the content of the preceding chapter applies to your personal experience. The journaling process is explored at greater length in chapter 10.

CHAPTER 6

◆

Dreams and Dream Interpretation

The interpretation of dreams is the royal road
to a knowledge of the unconscious activities
of the mind.

—SIGMUND FREUD,
The Interpretation of Dreams

————————————◆————————————

TEN MONTHS AFTER BILL'S DEATH
A cemetery visit triggers this dream

Bill and I arrive in our hotel room to attend a conference. Bill
says, *I have something to tell you; I'm leaving you.* He chokes
back tears but he's resolute. I struggle to compose myself. As
we leave the hotel, Bill asks if I remembered our research
poster, but I'm distraught and left it in our room.

In the dream, Bill doesn't look right and he's not behaving
normally. In life, he had an endearing disheveled look; in
the dream he's neat as a pin in his navy sport jacket and tan
pants, not a hair out of place, like a mannequin. His posture
is erect, his movements stiff, his behavior subdued.

We return to the hotel to retrieve the poster. Colleagues
are in our room. While I speak to others, Bill is mute and

motionless. I have a sudden urge to plead with him not to leave me. I reach for the rolled-up poster on the desk and knock the poster out of the open window. I watch it fall forty floors, tumbling end over end in slow motion. A luminous bride sees the poster falling and reaches out, catching it effortlessly; it floats right into her slender outstretched hand. I call out to her to recover the poster but my voice catches. I tell Bill to call out—he tries but his voice is weak, imperceptible. The radiant bride doesn't hear us and glides through a gate in a white picket fence carrying my poster.

COMMENT: *On awakening, I felt abandoned. It was the rare instance of verbal communication from Bill and it was painful. This sense of rejection obscured the other symbols in the dream for years, but now the content seems especially clear to me. The dream is singular since Bill speaks to me, announces he's leaving, reminds me of what I need to do, then recedes and withdraws. My early interpretation focused on Bill's departure in death, but years later I wonder if he's announcing his departure from my dreams, since he seldom appears again. I think I appear twice in this dream, as my current self and then as the bride. Initially, I cling to Bill as he prepares to leave, then I accept the baton as it's passed and glide through the gate, leaving an idyllic garden. Years later, the imagery of the ethereal bride and the poster drifting down those forty floors is vivid. Why forty? Only recently, I had a new thought: I turned 61 years old the year Bill died and was 21 when I first married . . . so, forty years had passed since I was a young bride. Was the dream traveling slowly back in time and then forward again, bridging the sense of abandonment with a vision of a new start?*

◆

Our emotional life and attachments, as intimate and substantial as they feel, stem from physical processes of the brain; they are generated by a vast network of neural transmission and signaling. And the pain and disorientation of traumatic loss is similarly a reflection of powerful neural imprints of memory and need. Every night, our thoughts and experiences are consolidated into long-term memory during the hours of sleep. Think of it like a filing system where new documents are initially placed in a short-term folder, to be carefully put away later and integrated with previous files (our past memories). This consolidation and reorganization of the new with the old is *the stuff that dreams are made of*—the mind's attempts to integrate new experiences into our preexisting understanding of our self and the world around us.

But what happens when the new experiences are traumatic—so strange and unfamiliar that they're unintelligible—*when your experience and your identity are incomprehensible to yourself?* A highly traumatic memory may be too disturbing to be integrated with past memory. This failure of integration with past memory often results in persistent unsettling dreams and prolonged emotional unrest.

Our dreams tend to reflect content from recent thoughts and experiences. Recurrent dreams featuring lost loved ones are common following a death or separation. After traumatic loss, some people stop remembering their dreams for months, while others begin to have unusually vivid dreams. Bereavement dreams come and go, and they may seem especially emotional and full of meaning. A painful experience may trigger a series of dreams; then months pass without any dreams. *When bereavement dreams are analyzed as a group over time—as a series of dreams following loss—they often reveal a progression of emotional adaptation and restoration.* In dream studies of people experiencing grief, 60% describe dreams of loved ones; most found these dreams to be pleasant, and few described having only disturbing dreams. Common dream themes include seeing loved ones restored to health or communicating a message. Disturbing themes include memories from times of illness and death.

The dissociative symptoms described in the previous chapter are transient disruptions in perception and awareness resulting from traumatic experience. Dissociation and other defense mechanisms are protective since they distance us from painful memories, but these defense mechanisms are also often associated with difficulty

REM sleep foster emotional restoration. Conversely, disrupted sleep, including insomnia, partial arousals, and nightmares, may block the healing process.

During sleep, the events of the day are integrated into deeper recesses of our mind by linking these recent experiences with similar past experiences. We can envision the vast complexity of this "filing system" where a single day's events link to previous memories of family, friends, work, mealtime, current events, books, and so on. Brain regions, including the *hippocampus* and *amygdala*, are involved in encoding emotional memories and generating dreams. During wakefulness, the amygdala is involved in expressing emotions and in dream recall; the amygdala is also one of the brain regions that is more active during REM sleep than during wakefulness. Problems occur when the indexing of memories is disrupted. A highly traumatic memory may be too disturbing to be integrated with other memories during REM sleep. People suffering from PTSD and prolonged grief aren't able to successfully consolidate traumatic memories; they experience persistent unsettling dreams and intrusive difficult memories when awake. This may in turn cause anxiety and *hypervigilance*, a condition in which emotions and memories (flashbacks) arise in response to various triggers. From a scientific perspective, dreams are internal traces of our memories and emotions.

DREAMS AS A SOURCE OF PERSONAL INSIGHT

The metaphorical stories dreams tell offer opportunities for moments of reflection and insight. Dr. Ullrich Wagner of the University of Munster studied the relationship between dreaming and insight with a mathematical task that can either be solved with lengthy calculations or by sudden insight into a hidden rule. Study participants were more than twice as likely to perceive the hidden rule after periods of sleep than after wakefulness. Brain fMRI, or functional MRI, is a technique for measuring brain activity by detecting changes in blood flow associated with neural activity. When fMRI was performed on the well-rested participants who perceived the shortcut based on the hidden rule, it showed greater activity in brain regions involved in memory, like the prefrontal cortex.

Neurophysiologist Matthew Walker developed another study paradigm that employed anagrams, or words formed by rearranging all of the letters of a different word or phrase (to give one example, rearranging the word *angel* to make the word *glean*). The study investigators found that people awakened during REM sleep solved more anagrams than people awakened during non-REM sleep or during the daytime, suggesting that REM sleep promotes cognitive flexibility and creativity. So sleep not only organizes and indexes memory, sleep aids in *developing fresh memory content* to foster emotional healing.

Emotional restoration reflects the gradual reorganization of memory traces at the level of our brain's neurons. This is called *neuroplasticity*—the remodeling of the brain's connections in response to experience. With time, these cumulative processes result in restructuring of our emotional responses and self-definition after traumatic loss. Many of us experience "aha" moments after a night's sleep, when a solution suddenly presents itself to a thorny problem. Creativity is increased upon awakening from REM sleep. Conversely, loss of sleep interferes with cognitive flexibility and finding solutions.

Mind wandering during wakefulness shares many similarities with dreaming; dreaming appears to be an intensified version of mind wandering. So, *daydreaming* is a pretty good term, more accurate and meaningful than we realize. While dreams may be longer, more visual, and immersive, mind wandering similarly involves complex integrations of emotions and memory that often result in problem-solving. Sleep, dreaming, and mind wandering are all important for emotional healing. This underscores the value of healthy sleep and pauses for meditation and reflection.

DREAMS AND DESENSITIZATION TO EMOTIONAL TRAUMA

Emotional memories are described as having two components: *memory content* and *emotional tone*. Dreams of lost loved ones may be comforting or disturbing. The dreamer may awaken feeling like they had contact with their loved one; dream content determines the emotional impact. Consolidating traumatic memories entails creating complex links with past memories that may result in cryptic, symbolic content.

REM sleep can be helpful because it strengthens memory content and weakens emotional tone. Greater clarity of recall and less emotional intensity fosters a new level of awareness. The metaphors of dreams may provide enough emotional distance from painful, threatening memories to enhance insight. For example, recalling emotional experiences of loss may be so highly charged that we're blocked from recalling these memories accurately—or even at all. Our mind may censor painful memories to protect us from further trauma. But dreams, journaling, and meditation result in gradual desensitization to the emotional charge, as well as gradual consolidation of traumatic experience. Important themes from these memories emerge as metaphors and symbols in our dreams, easing us into difficult territory. Our goal is to perceive our inner experience and gently raise awareness. Understanding the odd symbols in dreams is a process that happens over long periods of time, not just days and weeks, but months and years. Recording your dreams enables you to return to them periodically, reflecting on the strange stories once again, each time with greater insight.

After Bill's death, day and night journaling was triggered by my desire to search for answers, to understand what was happening to me. It seemed like dreams might be a portal to parts of my psyche that were inaccessible. I wondered, though: what approaches could I use to enhance insight into the content of my dreams?

THE CONTENT OF OUR DREAMS

Most dreams include bizarre elements, such as the merging of features of different people and places, and changes of these features across different dream sequences. However, dreams are also generally consistent with our waking experiences; for example, dreams rarely feature monsters or appear cartoonish.

Some other general comments about dreams: We appear in virtually all our own dreams. Dreams tend to feature our current concerns; they contain more emotional than situational content; and we nearly always interact with others during dreams. Also, dreams predominantly involve our visual and auditory senses; taste, smell, and tactile sensations are less common.

FIVE MONTHS AFTER BILL'S DEATH
An auditory dream

On two consecutive nights, I was awakened by a voice repeating my name over and over: *Lisa . . . Lisa . . . Lisa . . .* There was no dream sequence—only this auditory experience. It was a man's voice: kind and gentle, but unrecognizable. I awakened with the sense someone needed me.

THE ANNIVERSARY OF BILL'S DEATH
A tactile and auditory dream

I slept fitfully with thoughts of the anniversary at the forefront of my mind. Then I awakened with a start as I felt a tug on the bedclothes and heard someone slip under the sheets. I had the sense that a body slipped into the bed on Bill's side.

TYPES OF DREAMS FOLLOWING LOSS

Numerous surveys document the content of dreams experienced during grief, although these studies are limited by our capacity for dream recall. People who don't contemporaneously record their dreams are unlikely to recall them. Nonetheless, these surveys describe many common, recurring dream themes following loss. A 2003 article by Kathryn Belicki and colleagues examines the following themes:

Alive-Again or Back-to-Life: Loved ones reappear, often healthy and full of life.

Dying-Again: A replay of illness or end of life.

Saying-Goodbye: Appearance and departure; often, an affectionate goodbye.

Taking-a-Journey: Either the deceased or the survivor set out on a journey on a train, bus, or airplane. Common settings include airports and train or bus stations.

Communication or Advice-Comfort-Gift: Receiving a message from loved ones. A common message is *Don't worry, I'm fine.*

Approval-Disapproval: Loved ones show approval/disapproval of the survivor.

Passionate-Encounter: Loving and sensual encounters.

Daily-Activity: Later dreams with less emotional charge.

Taking–a-Journey comprised a disproportionate number of my dreams over the four years following Bill's death. These dreams were anxiety-provoking and had distinct recurring themes: traveling mishaps, lost baggage, lost tickets, no hotel reservations, disorientation and confusion.

◆

EIGHTEEN MONTHS AFTER BILL'S DEATH

I'm in an airport with my baggage on a cart. I have three pieces of baggage: two suitcases and a backpack. I'm concerned I'll misplace the baggage and I keep looking back at the cart to count the pieces. Sure enough, a suitcase goes missing! I feel foolish telling my son I've lost my suitcase. We scatter to search to no avail. Then my backpack is also gone. Again, searching ensues where I find an old backpack . . . not the one I lost. I'm at a loss for words about what's happening to me.

TWENTY-SIX MONTHS AFTER BILL'S DEATH
I'm having problems buying a ticket at the train station. The woman selling tickets ignores me and then leaves her desk. The train isn't coming so I take a bus to the airport and travel by air. I have no hotel reservations when I arrive, although I'm traveling to a meeting. I find a small bed and breakfast, but the owner and guests aren't welcoming; they're critical of my behavior. When I find the conference hotel, I plan to move my things, but I've brought too much. I have a trunk full of strange things—all sorts of unfamiliar jewelry and objects. I go through them one by one to decide what to keep and what to give away.

COMMENT: *The contrast between my waking life and my dream life is striking. In my waking life, I'm juggling the responsibilities of a practicing neurologist, researcher, and educator with frequent travel for business and family events—all with no difficulties. Yet in dream after dream, I'm utterly disorganized and unable to perform the most basic activities. This seems to capture the contrast between the structure and purposefulness of work and the sense of aimlessness in my personal life. Some dreams are odd and obscure, but these journey dreams are simple and prosaic—journeys to nowhere, losing baggage, unfamiliar belongings, no room at the inn . . . a lot of angst surrounding loss of identity and uncertainty for the future.*

Since we're all individuals with very different experiences, how can we explain why our dreams contain similar themes? Carl Jung, a Swiss psychiatrist and contemporary of Freud, described *archetypes* as collectively inherited unconscious ideas and patterns of thought that give rise to common, universal dream symbols. This suggests that the innate structure and function of our brain and mind give rise to shared patterns of thinking. This resonates with my experience as a neurologist caring for people with hallucinations and delusions in the setting of Parkinson's or Alzheimer's disease. Here again, common themes appear in patients' descriptions of their hallucinations and delusions. Commonly reported delusions, or false beliefs, include the conviction that a spouse is unfaithful or of being threatened or cheated. Common visual hallucinations include the reappearance of people or animals that have died or visions of bugs scurrying across the floor. In over twenty years of practice, I've yet to hear cheery hallucinations or delusions described, such as winning the lottery or relaxing on the beach. How can we explain this? These common neurologic phenomena are likely to reflect similarities in how we're hard-wired, how our brains are structured, and our evolutionary default to be vigilant to threats and danger.

So, as individual as the grief experience is, it's likely that some of these dream categories resonate with each of us. In addition to having dreams about taking a journey, my own dreams fit in the categories of Alive-Again and Communication. Dreams tend to vary with the time since the loss, the nature of the death, the stage of grief, and the relationship between you and your loved one.

J. William Worden, a psychologist at Harvard Medical School, proposed *tasks* of grief, in contrast to *stages*, to emphasize the effects of taking an active role in healing rather than passively moving through stages. These four tasks of grief are (1) to accept the reality of the loss, (2) to work through the pain of grief, (3) to adjust to an environment where our loved one is missing, and (4) to develop an enduring connection with our loved one and move on with our life. The content of dreams tends to evolve as we actively engage in each of these tasks. Studies of dream content over time show a gradual redefining of the relationship with our loved ones.

The dreams I recorded in my journal over four years following Bill's death show a progression through three phases. In the early dreams, Bill appears healthy, as he did before his illness. He is attentive and loving, but tends to appear suddenly, then disappear. In the intermediate dreams, there's a gradual change where Bill is increasingly stiff, robotic, indistinct, insubstantial, and mute. In the later, most recent dreams, Bill appears young, robust, and energetic, but more detached and aloof.

---------------------------------- ◆ ----------------------------------

FOUR YEARS AFTER BILL'S DEATH
Four sequences in one night

As I check out from a hotel, I see family members and join them to prepare a holiday dinner. I prepare dough for a challah, but leave the group as the bread rises. I feel lonely and distant.

Then I meet a friend who lost his wife. We prepare a simple breakfast—only tea.

Then Bill appears—he's young and energetic. He has a beard and a booming voice. He's in high spirits. He's cooking a big meal with gusto. I stop him to hold him close, and hesitantly describe how difficult it's been to be alone. He hugs me close—but fleetingly. He says, *I know*, and then he's back to cooking. Bill is reinvigorated and full of life, while I feel older and worn down. I've been changed by what's happened.

Bill and family reappear in the final dream sequence. Children and grandchildren scurry about while the women shop for clothes. The saleswoman displays an exotic outfit for me—a Native American motif with suede pants and a patterned sarong. Everyone likes it, including Bill. I think it's not what I need; I need more basic things.

COMMENT: *The dream juxtaposes the austere landscape of grief with the richness of family festivities. Bill is revitalized— full of life but distant. But years after his death, the inner work of integrating loss with the fullness of life continues. In each sequence, the final phrase offers important insights: I feel lonely and distant; I've been changed; I need more basic things.*

---------------------------------- ◆ ----------------------------------

DOCUMENTING AND INTERPRETING OUR DREAMS

When, in writing *The Interpretation of Dreams,* Freud cast about for
an analogy to describe the structure and shape of dreams, he found
it in the mushroom's mycelia, the membranous fibers that weave
together to form stalk and head, and that join together beneath
the earth to connect them with others of their kind. A dream,
like a mushroom, Freud thought, was an elaboration of its roots
in the past, in the tumult of unconscious feelings that sustained
and forced it into conscious awareness. And like a mushroom's
subterranean tendrils, a dream's dense layers of meaning were fused
and buried in the substratum of the dreamer's unconscious.

—MATTHEW VON UNWERTH, *Freud's Requiem: Mourning,*
Memory, and the Invisible History of a Summer Walk

After traumatic loss, we're challenged to grasp what happened to us, to
integrate this with our past, and to develop new levels of insight. Our
dreams are an important vehicle to meet these challenges. There's no
wrong way to interpret a dream since the meaning is deeply personal.
Over time, insights from the dream continue to change and evolve.
Keeping pen and paper on the bedside table is an important first step,
so that you can jot down your dreams and record new recollections
in the moment.

As I first scribble the content of a dream on waking from sleep,
the events never fail to seem strange and disjointed. Even the most
meaningful dreams appear trivial and senseless when I first jot them
down. The details of the dream come to me bit by bit; I never recall
the complete dream at first. Recall is triggered by reading and rereading my own words; waves of more detail drift back as I wash and
dress to start the day. I return again and again to the page to add
new information. Then at the end of the day, I return home to find
my scribbles on the dressing table. And as I read the dream story
again, it's oddly unfamiliar, like someone else wrote the whole thing.
Then memory returns and my mind is stirred once again to offer new
information and insights. I have learned the true value of recording
and interpreting dreams is this iterative process of investigation and

insight; this is more significant than finding *the true meaning* of the dream. This process comprises rich interludes of mindfulness, where bits and pieces of the unconscious are retrieved back into conscious awareness.

To understand our dreams, we should be attentive to many features: the setting, characters, story development, challenges, and the final event in the dream. This final event may reveal an unconscious solution to a problem or a key insight into the main theme. Most of the dream narratives found scattered through this book have significant final events. For example, in the dreams in this chapter, there is the sequence of the bride leaving the idyllic garden to pass through the gate, and there is the multi-sequence dream where I feel disconnected from festivities and conclude with the sense I've been changed; I need more basic things. In most dream sequences, the final event reveals a theme that clarifies previous events. At other times dreams simply dissolve at the end, possibly indicating that the meaning of events continues to be elusive. An example is found in the dream in the European inn, ending with my grandchild wandering into the next room.

Though dream content is often obscure, every setting and event in the dream is a glimpse into our inner world. Interpreting symbols in dreams can be tricky because they may have individual and unique meanings, yet there are also standard, shared symbols and metaphors that commonly appear. Since dreams are mostly visual, the unconscious mind uses visual images to express abstract concepts. Common themes include nakedness, taking a test, or finding new rooms in a house. Dream interpretation requires bridging the gap between these dream metaphors and our waking reality.

According to Carl Jung, the people in our dreams represent various aspects of ourselves. Therefore, we may appear as more than one character in the dream. This is interesting to thoughtfully consider, but also difficult to reconcile when familiar people appear in our dreams. Jung coined the term "the shadow" to describe a part of our unconscious where we hide features of ourselves we find distasteful or shameful. Jung believed that disturbing dreams and nightmares come from this shadow.

OBSCURE DREAMS VS. UNAMBIGUOUS DREAMS

The meaning of some dreams remains elusive, with symbols that are haunting and mysterious. Periodically, I return to these cryptic dreams to search for new insights. In contrast, other dreams are triggered by recent events and reflect unmistakable themes.

◆

TEN MONTHS AFTER BILL'S DEATH
After visiting the cemetery

I'm the bride in a wedding party. The groom is there, but indistinct, unrecognizable. The wedding planners instruct us to enter a small pool. There are five elderly people floating there, naked, pale, and inanimate. As we enter, two of the five reanimate and leave the pool to make room for us.

COMMENT: *The day of this dream, I visited the cemetery to check the installation of Bill's gravestone. In the twilight, I read the inscription engraved on the left side of the new gravestone out loud, and imagined my inscription on the right side of the stone. Then I traced a path between the row of graves, pausing to read each inscription and the names of the deceased. This disturbing dream depicts me descending into the pool with my husband, foreshadowing my own death.*

TWO YEARS AFTER BILL'S DEATH
After a memorial conference honoring Bill

I'm at a funeral. I've experienced a vast loss and people stop to comfort me. We're in a sculpture garden. People wander around the garden admiring the art and taking photos. The atmosphere is a strange mix, first lighthearted, then somber. At times, I sit sobbing alone. *Are we grieving for Bill? I'm not sure.* At one point, Bill appears; he doesn't speak but has a smile on his face to comfort me. Suddenly, there's a windstorm: the women's scarves wrap tightly around their faces.

You can no longer recognize them, but you see their features through the sheer scarves. People take photos of the veiled faces in the wind, and we laugh and laugh as we look at the images.

COMMENT: *These sequences describe the interface of personal and communal grief. The imagery of the veiled faces in the wind remains elusive, disturbing, and macabre. I believe the dream reveals the isolation of grief, my sense that others are masking their true feelings, and my desire to rejoin the community.*

◆

Loss and grief contain experiences so unfamiliar and jolting, there's often no way to connect them with past experience. There's no place to store these memories in the context of our lives. We must gradually make that place—a place where loss fits into our life experience—where it begins to make sense to us. This is the *raison d'être*—the purpose—of dreams, where new experiences are melded with old. With time, we witness signs of this transition in our daily life as we imperceptibly move from the inability to utter phrases like *he died* or *my home*, and begin to think and speak in terms of *my life* and *my future*. These are signs of progress and healing—signs of *Subconscious–Conscious Integration*.

By understanding our dreams, we gain a deeper understanding of ourselves and the world around us. Time spent reading and rereading my descriptions of dreams since Bill's death continues to be particularly meaningful. It's an unfiltered view of what's going on in my head, and the impact of these events in my life. As we work through grief, we're increasingly aware and mindful of the characteristics of our loved ones and their impact in our lives.

> Greater consciousness is the gift of death to the living
> who remain behind.
> —KYLE LEE WILLIAMS, "Dreams of Life and Death"

A PAUSE FOR JOURNALING

As you record your dreams and create a dream journal, peri-odically pause to thoughtfully review your descriptions, first, on the day of the dream, and then again days, weeks, months, and years later. Describe how you felt upon wakening and the emotions you experienced during the dream. Each time you review the dream, be open to new recollections and insights so you can elaborate on the events and the meanings. This may involve editing the dream, rewriting the dream, or adding commentary.

- Look for images and symbols that spur elaboration and interpretation. What associations and memories do the symbols bring to mind?
- Rereading the dream may stir up emotions; be sensitive to these emotions and express them in your writing. Record when you sense you've connected to a deeper meaning.
- You may find the content of a dream completely obscure. It may be too soon for you to connect with the dream symbols and metaphors. With time, the contents of the dream may gradually reveal themselves.
- Reflect on each dream in the context of other dreams and over the span of time. Date each dream so you can search for evolving themes.

CHAPTER 7

•

The Science of the Wounded Mind

> ... although mourning involves grave departures from
> the normal attitude toward life, it never occurs to us
> to regard it as a pathological condition and to refer it
> to a medical treatment. We rely on its being overcome
> after a certain lapse of time, and we look upon any
> interference with it as useless or even harmful.
> —SIGMUND FREUD, *Mourning and Melancholia*

GRIEF IS JARRING. Beset by unfamiliar emotions, we may question if we're losing our mind. As time goes by after loss, we're discouraged by emotional setbacks, and it may seem like a sign of weakness when we're distressed or tearful years later. But think about the gradual healing process of a broken bone or a wound following surgery. After physical injury, it doesn't seem surprising that people heal at different rates or that unfortunate circumstances may delay healing. Yet when we reflect on healing after loss, it can be hard to imagine that we'll ever feel whole again, no less be all the wiser after difficult times.

A century ago, Sigmund Freud described grief as a serious but normal emotional process following the death of a loved one. Freud was mainly concerned with the distinction between grief and severe depression, which he called melancholia. And although Freud also studied the psychiatric effects of traumatic events, he viewed the experiences of grief and trauma as wholly different problems.

Many studies of emotional trauma grew out of combat experiences during the First and Second World Wars and the Vietnam War, resulting in a continued separation of views on grief and trauma during most of the twentieth century. The last two decades have seen a large shift of opinion, with growing consensus about the presence of more prolonged forms of grief and mounting controversy related to the similarities and differences between grief and trauma.

Two psychologists with extensive expertise in bereavement, Lauren Breen and Mary-Frances O'Connor, describe a basic paradox in the grief literature. On the one hand, they point out, every grief experience is unique, based on many personal and situational factors. On the other hand, there's increasing consensus in differentiating *common grief* from *complicated grief* based on certain symptoms and time frames. The paradox lies in the simultaneous recognition of vast individual differences between people dealing with loss, yet the common impulse to find a clear distinction between normal vs. abnormal adjustment. How can we make sense of the experience of loss in a person in particularly adverse personal circumstances? Is their prolonged grief an expected outcome of especially difficult circumstances, or is their delayed recovery a sign of poor adjustment?

There are many pervasive assumptions about grief embedded in our culture and in scholarly literature. Conventional wisdom holds that grief follows a distinct pattern, proceeds in stages, and is short-term and finite. It's commonly believed that successful grief work results in resolution and that prolonged grief is deviant. If we are slow to heal, we're likely to judge ourselves harshly. We may question whether our behavior is extreme or whether our progress is inadequate. Importantly, we may turn away from our instinct to do things that comfort us in the belief that there are right and wrong ways to behave.

Cultural guideposts and mental health specialists may endorse prevailing beliefs in accepted timelines, stages of grief, and an expectation of *closure*, thereby creating a belief that continued bonds to loved ones are abnormal. But our experience of loss is personal and intimate. It doesn't lend itself well to generalization; it's as unique as we are. And while our circumstances are different, we can learn from each other's experiences. We each find our own way of sustaining bonds to our loved ones, like when I wrap myself up in Bill's soft woolen scarf on a cold, windy day. The tie that binds us together is the performance of these rituals and the comfort they continue to bring. There's value in listening to instinct and in becoming a keen observer of what brings comfort and what results in heightened distress.

Clinicians and researchers are drawn to categorization. Whether the problem is asthma, diabetes, epilepsy, or my own field, Parkinson's disease, classification serves an important purpose, even though we often see patients and phenomena that don't neatly fit into our attempts to create order. Without grouping and labeling, there would be no common vocabulary for clinicians to discuss their patients' problems and no way for researchers to group patients with similar problems to investigate new treatments. For example, the psychologist needs to describe their patient's condition in a way that the primary care physician will understand. And when the researcher describes a study comparing people with symptoms of *common grief* to people with *prolonged grief,* the community of bereavement researchers needs to be on the same page. Nonetheless, the range and depth of individual experience can never be captured in neat categories of diagnostic subgroups. This is surprisingly true for both medical and psychiatric conditions.

When it comes to individual approaches to classification, clinicians often describe themselves as either *lumpers* or *splitters*. Lumpers tend to see similarities between subgroups and instinctively create larger categories with similar phenomena. Splitters tend to see differences between subgroups and intuitively create smaller categories based on detailed criteria. These philosophical differences in approach give rise to controversy: Is grief in all its manifestations simply a normal response, or should some types of grief be "pathologized" and considered mental health disorders? Are traumatic loss and post-traumatic stress umbrella terms that include all types of painful loss (bereavement, divorce, new medical diagnosis, natural disasters, physical assault), or is bereavement fundamentally different from other forms of traumatic stress?

Lance P. Kelley, a psychologist at Auburn University, compared post-traumatic symptoms between people with grief to others who experienced a motor vehicle accident or sexual assault. Post-traumatic symptoms were observed in all three conditions, with the greatest severity following sexual assault followed by grief and then motor vehicle accident. These results support the notion that post-traumatic stress is a final common pathway with many portals of entry.

What differentiates bereavement from a traumatic event? Some experts limit the definition of trauma to only include violent or untimely events, but this repudiates many common experiences of traumatic loss, such as when someone who is integral to our identity dies following illness. For example, the expected and timely death of a beloved elderly person frequently results in traumatic loss for their spouse, even when death is anticipated. *The traumatic nature of events lies in their personal meaning.* And personal meaning will encompass a vast range of losses. Not all grief is traumatic, and not all trauma involves bereavement, but the two concepts strongly overlap.

Whether you're a lumper or a splitter, categorization requires descriptive criteria. Lines must be drawn somewhere. But these lines fail to capture the granularity and texture of human experience. This problem is illustrated in the psychiatrist's "bible" for classifying mental disorders known as the *DSM–5* (the *Diagnostic and Statistical Manual of Mental Disorders*, fifth edition). This latest edition added criteria to differentiate grief from prolonged, complicated grief. Nearly 15 million people in the United States experience grief at any one time, and between 10 to 20% of people with bereavement develop complicated grief. The *DSM–5* also revised its criteria for PTSD, expanding the number of common symptoms people experience following traumatic stress. Notably, by recognizing more symptoms of traumatic stress, the manual has significantly increased the number of permutations of symptoms that cause doctors to arrive at a PTSD diagnosis. This point was brought home by Isaac Galatzer-Levy and Richard Bryant in their 2013 paper, "636,120 Ways to Have Posttraumatic Stress Disorder," which calculated there are 636,120 possible symptom combinations! Ironically, broadening PTSD classification by adding precise diagnostic criteria has the unintended effect of producing ambiguous results due to excessive detail.

A person's risk of developing prolonged grief, PTSD, or other emotional problems is influenced by many factors, including his or her personality, social network, and genetics. There are three categories of *risk factors* for greater problems with adjustment: *situational* (perception of events surrounding the illness and death), *personal* (personality, gender, poor health), and *interpersonal* (social support, finances). Risk factors are also known as *susceptibility factors*. They include the circumstances of the death (was it anticipated, violent, or following a long illness?), the quality of a person's relationship with the person who dies, and the characteristics of the person grieving, including their age, gender, coping style, and life history.

Psychologists also recognize that genetics plays a significant role in emotional adjustment and psychiatric disorders. Psychologist Mark W. Gilbertson conducted a fascinating study of trauma that compared forty pairs of identical twins. One twin in each pair had been exposed to combat. Close to half of those who had fought in combat developed PTSD; MRI imaging showed that the size of the brain region known as the *hippocampus* was unusually small in those who developed the disorder. Intriguingly, the study found that the twin who hadn't experienced combat *also had a small hippocampus* (but didn't have PTSD). This suggests that a small hippocampus is a risk factor, or a sign of greater vulnerability, for developing PTSD following stressful experiences. This study shows how *both genetic factors and life events combine to create vulnerability.* Understanding our personal vulnerabilities and risks helps us cope and adapt. Insight into our individual situations is empowering, enabling us to be mindful and effective in managing grief.

Just as each of us has a *risk profile* of our capacity to manage traumatic loss, we also have a *resilience profile*. Resilience is our ability to successfully adapt and recover when we experience life's adversities. Resilience may include not only recovery, but also psychological growth following trauma. Greater resilience is seen in people with childhood experiences that fostered security and safety, a tendency to experience positive emotions like well-being and optimism, and a sense of meaning and purpose in life. Purpose in life may come from many sources, including family, career, mindfulness, religion, or spirituality. Resilience is also enhanced by the belief that we influence what happens in our lives, as well as the ability to learn from both positive and negative experiences. Resilient people are more likely to be comforted by thinking about their loved ones and less likely to search for meaning in their death.

Returning to the lumpers and splitters, it's not clear whether there are two distinct categories of people with *grief* vs. *complicated grief.* The *DSM–5* describes complicated grief (also called prolonged grief or traumatic grief) as being characterized by symptoms of intense yearning and loneliness, futility about the future, feeling like life is meaningless, or having the sense that a part of us has died. Complicated grief is also defined by persistent, intense grief symptoms six months following the loss of a loved one.

But let's be sensible: grief is experienced in waves, it waxes and wanes, and it's not watching the calendar. There are inevitable reminders and other triggers that increase grief, some predictable (birthdays, anniversaries, holidays) and some totally unexpected. Grief symptoms may overlap with anxiety, depression, and sleep disorders. There's a tendency to be too quick to pathologize the broad range of responses to diverse circumstances of trauma. Experiencing a loss of identity, dissociating, or adopting habits of the deceased may all sound extreme, but the experience of traumatic loss *is* extreme. Grief symptoms are best judged based on whether behavior relieves suffering, sustains daily function, and promotes gradual restoration of balance and equanimity. If there's a threshold of excessive grief, should there also be a threshold for too little? Taking a more impartial view of human response to loss may be more sensible, one in which grief is considered unhealthy when the response appears disproportionate to the loss or disrupts the ability to function.

When people complete a grief inventory—a questionnaire that surveys grief symptoms—respondents suffering from a loss continue to report symptoms for not just months, but for years and sometimes indefinitely. After ten years, the most commonly endorsed grief inventory items included "No one will ever take his/her place in my life," "At times I still feel that I need to cry for him/her," and "At times I feel as though he/she is still with me."

Neuropsychotherapist and bereavement expert Dr. Judith Murray draws the distinction between integration of loss and resolution of loss, where *the healthy process of grief involves continuing bonds that survivors maintain with the deceased*. She describes integrated grief as an ongoing process where emotional healing and restoration are underway, even though the bereaved is forever changed by the loss. There's comfort in knowing that our relationships with loved ones endure, that this is normal and expected, and that there's no time limit on these sacred bonds.

As a neurologist, I find that the metaphor of the wounded mind and brain makes sense. We understand the concept of a wound healing. The healing process goes through stages that may be shorter or longer in different people. When medical doctors assess the healing process of a physical wound, our main focus is whether healing is continuing. Do we observe reassuring signs of progress, or signs of emerging problems that will retard healing? When we judge whether the process is proceeding abnormally or taking too long, we consider many factors. How serious was the wound? What is the age and health of the patient? Did the person reinjure themselves in the course of the healing process? Is normal scar tissue forming, or are there signs of infection where the wound appears increasingly angry and painful? When the wound doesn't heal or even worsens over time, it needs medical attention. But when the wound gradually improves—understandably slowly in some circumstances—and the person gradually regains function, we perceive this as part of a natural healing process.

Why not judge the grief process through the same lens?

Again, *the traumatic nature of events lies in their personal meaning*. The severity of each loss is personal, and a person's healing process will vary based on many individual factors. Extending this analogy, when a wound is especially severe, we may not expect things to go back to the way they were. Healing will run its course, but scars will remain and rehabilitation, or counseling, may be necessary to help the person optimize their function by learning to live with this loss.

Similarly, there are times when recovery from grief stalls or we're disabled by grief and need the assistance of professionals.

Mary-Frances O'Connor, an associate professor of clinical psychology at the University of Arizona, poses a pivotal question about recovery following traumatic loss. Do we return to our previous baseline function following a period of grief? Or does grief result in a learning process—which she calls *stress-related growth*—that results in a new way of functioning? Traumatic loss results in disruption of our identity—how we see ourselves. Do we restore our baseline identity or rebuild and reconstruct the narrative of our lives? There's a natural instinct to make sense of what happens to us; when life feels random and unpredictable, it's difficult to set goals and make plans. When people experience trauma, they sense unpredictability in the world. Recovery involves finding a new balance, where we build confidence in what lies ahead and belief in our ability to handle adversity so we can gradually regain our bearings.

A Pause for Journaling

The traumatic nature of events lies in their personal meaning. Describe the personal meaning of this loss. Then describe your personal balance of risk and resilience factors in response to traumatic loss, recalling the three categories of risk factors: *situational* (perception of events surrounding the illness and death), *personal* (personality, gender, poor health), and *interpersonal* (social support, finances). Remember that risk factors also include the circumstances of the death (anticipated, violent, following a long illness), the quality of the relationship with the person who dies, and the characteristics of the person grieving including their age, gender, coping style, and previous life history.

CHAPTER 8

•

The Science of the Wounded Brain

Our individual experiences of loss are so textured, so layered with meaning—it strains credulity that there could be a scientific, corporeal explanation for these vivid emotional experiences. But as knowledge of the workings of the mind, brain, and body deepens, we increasingly understand how brain science explains emotions of grief and loss. Simply put, psychiatry and neurology are the same thing. All of our emotions and behavior, indeed the totality of our experience, has a neurologic basis. It's not possible to separate the yearning and loneliness of grief from the biologic effects of emotional trauma on the brain.

Experiencing traumatic loss—witnessing the suffering and death of loved ones—is harrowing. This chapter describes how emotional stress and the function of mind, brain, and body are closely connected.

How Our Bodies Respond to the Stress of Grief

To ensure survival, our mind, brain, and body are hard-wired to respond rapidly to stress. These responses are designed to help us react to threats, adapt to challenges, and learn from experience, so that in the end, we're safe and all the wiser. It's not at all surprising that stress results in widespread effects throughout the body. Stress is a strong promoter of *neuroplasticity,* the brain's capacity to be dynamic and adaptive—to develop new neurons and to remodel neural connections.

A brief description of the *stress response mechanism* is important to understand the effects of grief on our body. Although designed to adapt to threats, stress-induced changes can result in either a return to health and homeostasis or to maladaptation. In fact, chronic persistent stress and depression can disrupt the neuroplasticity needed for healing. In contrast, stress reduction can enhance neural recovery. In other words, stress results in a cascade of body changes that may either lead to restoration and recovery or to enduring problems, including anxiety, depression, or PTSD.

The stress response has two main parts: the rapid *fight-or-flight* response and the longer stage of *recovery and adaptation.* Briefly, stress activates the brain's *hypothalamus,* which initiates the fight-or-flight response. Hormones—*adrenaline* and *cortisol*—are released to sound the alarm: *Heads up! Risk, threat, danger!* Adrenaline increases heart rate, blood pressure, and respiratory rate—vital for fight-or-flight; cortisol enhances memory and adjustment to stressful events. This stress cascade is the key link between stress and its pervasive effects on the mind, brain, and body—with different consequences when the stress is fleeting (encountering a bear on a hike) than when it's enduring (traumatic loss and grief).

Takotsubo syndrome, also known as broken heart syndrome, is a vivid example of the mind-brain-body connection. People suffering from takotsubo syndrome, which was first described in 1990, experience an amplified response to severe stress. Stressful events activate the fight-or-flight hormones, causing abnormal movement of the heart muscle and resulting in typical symptoms of heart attack: chest pain and shortness of breath. These symptoms are usually transient and reversible, since there's no accompanying build-up of plaque or narrowing of blood vessels to the heart. However, intensely stressful experiences can result in actual injury to the heart muscle. The syndrome gets its name from the takotsubo pot, an octopus trap used by Japanese fishermen; the earliest descriptions of this syndrome compared the ballooning shape of the heart's ventricle to the shape of

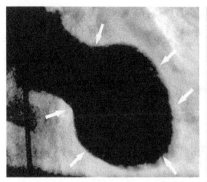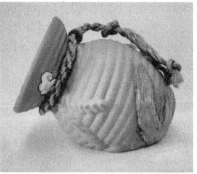

Ballooning of the ventricle of the heart (*left*) resembles the shape of the Japanese takotsubo pot, an octopus trap used by Japanese fishermen.

the pot. Takotsubo predominantly affects older women, but may also occur in men and among younger people.

There are recent reports of people simultaneously experiencing both takotsubo syndrome and a second syndrome, *transient global amnesia*. Transient global amnesia is a reversible brain disorder characterized by sudden memory loss for recent events. People suffering from this type of amnesia often ask repetitive questions; they sound like broken records, so to speak. As with takotsubo syndrome, episodes of transient global amnesia are triggered by stressful experiences and associated with the activation of fight-or-flight hormones. This is a vivid example of mind-brain-body interactions.

Neuroimaging

The development of sensitive and precise tools for brain imaging is advancing understanding of mind-brain connections. Magnetic resonance imaging (MRI) scanning results in exquisitely detailed images of brain structures. More recently, functional MRI (fMRI) reveals a combination of both brain *structure and function* by measuring activity in specific areas of the brain. Valuable insights arise from comparing fMRI images of brain structure and function between different groups of people: for example, people who are grieving versus not grieving, as well as people who are happy and people who are sad. Researchers also administer mental tasks to people experiencing grief in order to study the difference between people actively remembering loss versus being distracted from thoughts of loss.

A review of eighteen fMRI studies of brain areas affected by painful emotions identified a neural network—comprising inter-connected pathways that are activated by painful emotions—that includes these key areas: the *cerebellum, cingulate cortex, parahippo-campal gyrus,* and *thalamus.* These brain areas overlap with regions of the brain that are activated during physical pain. Neural pathways involved in regulating attention during grief are also important, since daily function at home or at work depends upon the ability to suppress intrusive thoughts of loss. fMRI scans show that activity and connectivity between the brain's *amygdala* and *prefrontal cortex* are associated with better regulation of attention during grief. These studies reveal the intimate relationships between emotional trauma and brain function.

The amygdala plays an especially pivotal role in our response to trauma by coding both the intensity and *valence,* or relative positive vs. negative value, of emotions. The valence or value refers to levels of positive emotions such as joy and well-being, or negative emotions such as fear and sorrow. Essentially, the amygdala regulates our per-ception of vulnerability and threat and thereby also regulates our capacity to make sound life decisions.

A well-known example is *Pavlovian fear conditioning.* This classic experiment paired a neutral conditioned stimulus, like an auditory tone, with an *unconditioned stimulus*: a painful or threatening con-dition that naturally results in a stress response. When a neutral, nonthreatening stimulus (the sound of a bell) is paired with an actual threat (like a foot shock), the neutral stimulus becomes associated with pain and is then called the *conditioned stimulus.* Accordingly, when rodents are exposed to several repetitions of both stimuli, the neutral stimulus (the tone) elicits the fight-or-flight response *with-out* the painful stimulus (the shock). This is the amygdala at work, incorrectly calibrating the threat of the harmless tone and sparking a disproportionate emotional response, not unlike our exaggerated emo-tional response to many triggers after trauma. Notably, the Pavlovian model also shows the capacity for *fear extinction*—an active learning process where repeated exposure to only the trigger (the neutral stimulus) gradually disconnects the harmless trigger from the painful stimulus. This is an example of neuroplasticity and learning, where neuronal connections are remodeled based on new experience. Therefore, to promote emotional healing, we seek to thoughtfully uncouple emotional pain and threat from our treasured memories.

Brain Areas Activated during Grieving

BRAIN REGION	DESCRIPTION OF FUNCTION
Amygdala	Involved in emotion and memory, including fear, separation anxiety, and arousal
Cerebellum	Associated with coordination and balance; more recently linked to emotions and cognition
Cingulate Cortex	Involved in interactions between emotion and memory (emotional responses, impulse control, decision-making) and autonomic functions (blood pressure, heart rate)
Hippocampus	Plays an important role in consolidating short-term memories into long-term memories
Hypothalamus	Links the nervous system to the hormonal system; important regulator of fatigue, sleep, circadian rhythms, hunger, thirst, body temperature, and attachment
Limbic System	The *emotional brain* containing the amygdala, hippocampus, hypothalamus, and thalamus
Parahippocampal Gyrus	Surrounds the hippocampus; involved in memory, including recognition of places, situations, and social context
Prefrontal Cortex	Involved in complex behaviors, including personality, social behaviors, and decision-making
Thalamus	A key relay station connecting the cerebral cortex (which makes us aware of emotions, enabling us to be introspective and to draw insights) with nearly all brain regions

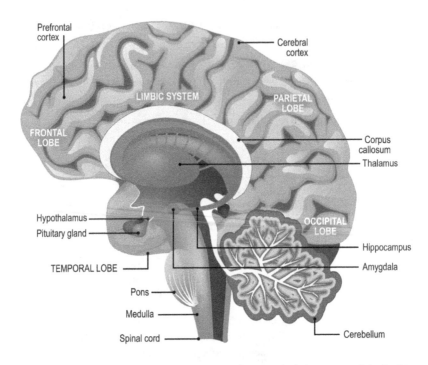

Brain regions affected by stress and emotional pain include key areas of the limbic system: the amygdala, hippocampus, hypothalamus, and thalamus.

O'Connor developed an intriguing paradigm to investigate brain regions activated during grieving. Bereaved participants were exposed to four study conditions during fMRI: (1) a photo of the person who died + written grief-related words, (2) a photo of the person who died + neutral words, (3) a photo of a stranger + grief-related words, and (4) a photo of a stranger + neutral words. Simultaneously, participants' skin conductance—the electrical conductance of the skin, which varies depending on the level of moisture—was monitored. Since skin moisture increases during the fight-or-flight response, skin conductance can be used as a measure of emotional response. The results showed that the most intense brain activation was elicited by the first set of conditions—the photo of the person who died + grief-related words—and the smallest brain response was elicited by the fourth set of conditions, the photo of a stranger + neutral words. The second and third sets of conditions elicited intermediate brain responses. This paradigm teases apart the impact of visual imagery compared to written words, showing that different areas of the brain are activated based on grief-related pictures versus words. This study model also clearly demonstrates mind-brain-body connections, as the skin conductance response (fight-or-flight arousal) varied with the intensity of grief reminders.

Like all behavior, the human capacity to form strong enduring relationships is grounded in mechanisms of brain function. Studies of romantic love and sexual attraction show that these emotions activate reward centers in the brain that are regulated by dopamine and other transmitters. Brain activity patterns from fMRI are remarkably similar in (a) people viewing photos of romantic partners, (b) mothers viewing images of their children, and (c) people receiving cocaine or opioid infusions. These unlikely associations show that close social attachments and addiction share neural mechanisms that involve the reward center of the brain, and suggest parallels between the physical pain of addictive drug withdrawal and the emotional pain of traumatic loss. Therefore, disruption of strong social bonds, as is caused by divorce or the death of loved ones, results in anxiety, agitation, and pain due to the breakdown of healthy brain function.

The Brain and Behavior: Lessons from Neurosurgery

Deep brain stimulation is a well-recognized neurosurgical procedure in which electrodes are implanted deep within the brain. Electrical stimulation results in modulation of the targeted neural pathways. This procedure is approved for use in patients with Parkinson's disease and is now under investigation for psychiatric problems, including depression and obsessive-compulsive disorder. Like many medical discoveries, the first clues that electrical stimulation of the brain induced changes of emotion were serendipitous. Doctors and researchers observed that postoperative stimulation of electrodes induced sudden feelings of sadness, guilt, and hopelessness in patients following this procedure. Now, there are numerous reports documenting the induction of varied emotions during deep brain stimulation procedures, ranging from anxiety and depression to calmness, improved mood, and euphoria. It's both fascinating and unsettling to perceive the intimate relationship between our brain's neural circuitry and our emotions and behavior.

Brain and Body Connections

Hormones

Cortisol, one of those fight-or-flight hormones, is normally at peak levels when we wake up in the morning and then rapidly falls as the day progresses. Stress disrupts this cycle, causing abnormally low morning cortisol levels and abnormally high levels throughout the day. When a study compared daily cortisol levels in people with depression associated with grieving vs. people with depression that was not associated with grief, only the grieving group had abnormal cortisol levels. Furthermore, cortisol regulation was more abnormal in people who had more recently lost a loved one. This study also found that elevated cortisol and adrenaline levels following loss predicted greater hopelessness, poorer health, and a higher frequency of hospitalization one year following loss.

Yet another study showed faster heart rates in people experiencing grief than people with non-grief-induced depression or in a non-depressed control group. Surprisingly, among the grieving group, a faster heart rate in the early weeks after loss predicted *earlier* adjustment a year later. This outcome echoes the process of stress-neuroplasticity-adaptation, where the stress response (manifested by increased heart rate) promotes remodeling of neural pathways and facilitates healthy adjustment over time. In summary, hormonal changes triggered by traumatic loss result in emotional and physical symptoms that are normal and necessary for healthy recovery.

Immune System Function

The previously described fMRI paradigm that presented subjects with four sets of pictures and words was also used to study whether grieving is associated with inflammation and immune dysfunction. The results show that grief not only activates key brain pathways, but increases inflammation in the body. In short, bereavement may cause dysfunction of the immune system. The immune system controls our body's response to injury and disease, including the inflammatory response. We commonly observe inflammation, such as redness and swelling, of an infected skin wound; this is the normal immune response to fight infection. During bereavement, blood tests show poor function of immune cells, which may result in an increased risk of illness following emotional trauma. Importantly, this disruption of immune function isn't likely to have major consequences in people who are healthy, but may be more consequential in people with pre-existing health problems, especially disorders of the immune system.

Sleep

Traumatic loss causes disturbed sleep, including trouble falling asleep and maintaining sleep. This is related to excessive activation of sleep-related brain centers, including the amygdala, an important mediator of arousal, fear, and anxiety. In a vicious cycle, activation of brain centers of arousal causes insomnia following traumatic loss, and this insomnia prolongs stress-related arousal. In the same way that cortisol regulation is disrupted by loss, another hormone—*melatonin*—may also be affected and contribute to sleep disturbance. Melatonin is normally produced close to bedtime and is involved in circadian rhythms and timing of sleep.

TRAUMATIC LOSS AND GRIEF result in important and measurable changes across many body systems, exemplified by effects on hormonal regulation, the immune response, and sleep. Increased morbidity and mortality—in other words, illness and death from all causes—are associated with grief. Nonetheless, the link between bereavement and the development and progression of disease remains controversial. Understanding the pervasive biologic effects of traumatic loss on our health and function, underscores the importance of taking proactive steps to foster healing.

As we review the science of grief, we acknowledge these studies are complex and have limitations. It's never straightforward to firmly answer any scientific question. For example, study subjects experiencing grief vary in terms of the time since their loss, the type of loss, their individual personalities, and their overall health. When rating grief severity, the actual time since the death of a loved one may not be as important as a person's individual progress with coping and adjustment. These limitations confound the results of all studies and highlight the importance of our individual experience.

It's important to draw a distinction between normal protective stress responses and dysfunction resulting in physical or mental health problems. For instance, the amygdala of the brain is involved in recognizing and modulating attention to fearful experiences. These are evolutionary protective functions, harkening back to the need to be vigilant to predators—to develop instincts to avoid life-threatening situations. Psychologists David M. Diamond and Phillip R. Zoladz compared the ramped-up function of the amygdala to *a bull in the evolutionary china shop*. Thinking literally, we can envision the bull wreaking havoc in the china shop, but from the bull's perspective, he just wants to protect himself and get out of there. Similarly, the person experiencing traumatic loss has survived a crisis, a life-threatening event. Brain centers involved in stress and fear are hyperfunctional and sensitized to the next threat. This condition of high alert represents a turning point where healthy adjustment will reduce the sense of danger, calming the bull in the china shop and restoring a safe environment. If healthy adjustment is impossible, the fear system remains in overdrive, and we exhibit the symptoms of hyperarousal, depression, and sleep problems seen in PTSD.

Stress can have both positive and negative effects. Since stress is one of the most potent triggers for neuroplasticity, stressful times are fertile opportunities for either growth or maladaptation. Optimal stress levels can drive people to acquire new skills, whereas extreme chronic stress can lead to persistent emotional problems. *Since grief and loss can't be avoided, how can we manage stress to increase our potential for growth and reduce the risk of maladaptation?*

The goal is clear: people suffering from grief need to encourage the protective benefits of stress and avoid the harmful effects. We need to be mindful of the need to promote healthy adjustment. We need to be purposeful in making life choices that enhance adaptation and nudge us gently on the right path. We need to seek the right balance of periods of distraction, where the mind can rest, and periods of mindful meditation, where we recall our difficulties. This balance is expressed in the second principle of healing, *Immersion–Distraction*. In this way, we consolidate the stressful memories gradually, at our own pace. There are many active things we can do to find this balance, including journaling, undergoing counseling, and reading to reflect on our experience of loss. Work, hobbies, and exercise are opportunities to focus energy in new areas and take a needed rest from grief and mourning. With time, these immersive and distracting activities need to be adjusted to complement evolving emotional healing and restoration.

Close interpersonal relationships are core components of *who we are*. The loss of people closest to us results in unanticipated emotional trauma—a disorganization and disruption of our identity. Seeing emotional trauma as a form of stress-related injury to the mind, brain, and body is important, and is too often deemphasized in America's cultural interpretation of grief.

As I walk the line between my own experience of bereavement and my background in neuroscience, I confess my "scientist hat" doesn't always fit quite as snugly as usual. Instead, this hat is cocked to one side, leaving room for special moments that defy explanation and bring comfort.

We needn't choose—we can find room for both scientific and spiritual understanding of our experiences. After Bill was gone, his daughter asked, *Aren't you kind of waiting for a pigeon to light on your shoulder and wink at you?* Even a scientist can warm to that image.

A Pause for Journaling

Describe your own approach to *immersion* and *distraction*. Are you finding a balance between periods of distraction (where the mind can rest) and periods of mindfulness (where we recall our difficulties)? Does your approach promote the health of your mind, brain, and body? Review key health indicators, including your energy level, physical activity, sleep habits, and the stability of your medical conditions.

HEALING AND RESTORATION

CHAPTER 9

•

Developing Confidence
in Managing Grief and Loss

....

Dear Bill,

You've been gone ten months. You taught me about mindfulness—
being present in the moment. You made it appear effortless. Where
I'm goal-oriented, you were about process. Where I dwell on what
may go wrong, you dropped little notes in my lunch bag saying
"Things will go well." Where I ruminate over blunders, you were
easy on yourself and forgiving. You showed grace in accepting
what life brings—even during the worst of times.

I witnessed this grace: the quiet absorption you brought to
simple tasks; how you cut and mixed ingredients when preparing
dinner; how you slowly removed your glasses to inspect details of
a hand-crafted piece. And there was spontaneity as you followed
whims to pore over books in our library. Life's annoyances man-
aged without undue angst. With you by my side, I was carried
along by these natural flowing currents. Left to my own instincts,
I default to assembling to-do lists and Post-it notes. A redundant
set of reminders and alerts, so lists are literally in my face. Really,
will the world come to an end if I forget something? It's mindful-
ness I'm seeking, not reminaholfulness.

So here's the problem: You were my GPS. I found mindfulness
with you, where the noise of the world was tamed, where our
home was a sanctuary. You showed how clarity and peace of mind
comes from within. Now I take my first steps on this path alone.
Shadowing you, I pause at our window to watch autumn foliage
turn to naked branches etched by winter's frost. And I'm easier
on myself—so I can venture out and take risks. And as I walk in
your footsteps, I feel comforted. Confronting loss and loneliness,
the antidote appears to be connectivity—but I sense the path to
healing is within.

How would things go if our positions were reversed—if I
were gone and you were alone? How would you spend your time?
Would you find companionship? Would our bond be both comfort
and obstacle: the comfort of what was and the obstacle to move
forward? And for a few moments, I imagine escape from this
alien world.

LOSS OF A LIFE PARTNER leaves us isolated and exposed. Loss of
cherished family or friends leaves us with a heavy sense of isolation.
Others may not understand the impact of these personal losses. At
times, grief rises up and threatens to swallow us whole, yet even at its
worst, we glimpse that this time in our lives will compel us to search
deep inside and learn about ourselves. In the first weeks after Bill
was gone, I described to a wise elder my sense of being enveloped by
an eerie solitude. *At the end of the day, aren't we all really alone?* he
asked. Initially, I was stunned; horrified. But a small inner voice knew
he was right.

The psychiatrist Irvin Yalom described two kinds of loneliness,
everyday and *existential*. Everyday loneliness is the pain of literally
being isolated from others.

> The second form of loneliness, existential isolation,
> is more profound and stems from the unbridgeable gap
> between the individual and other people. This gap is a
> consequence not only of each of us having been thrown

alone into existence and having to exit alone, but
derives from the fact that each of us inhabits a world
fully known only to ourselves.
—IRVIN D. YALOM, *Staring at the Sun:*
Overcoming the Terror of Death

Traumatic loss exposes the reality that life is not within our control. This truth is softened by recognizing the universality of loss in human experience. We're surrounded by people who experience similar challenges. Many forms of Eastern spirituality teach followers to find peace by accepting life as it is: unconditionally. According to an article by Dr. Cecilia Chan and colleagues, we can manage the impasse between our sense of control and reality *by distinguishing control over life choices in response to life events, from control over life events*. When we're consumed by the loss of what we had planned for our future, we're unable to see possibilities around us. My own perspective shifted when I stumbled on this thought in Tamar Adler's *New York Times Magazine* story, "The Taste of Serendipity": *If you're not looking for things to be perfect, you can see more of what's there.* This sage advice applies, even though it was used to describe conquering the challenge of preparing a recipe when the precise ingredients are missing!

Does the inner work of grief result in better outcomes, including *post-traumatic growth*—the experience of positive change as a result of struggling with highly challenging life crises? *Heightened existential awareness*—which involves examining life more deeply— has been found to improve post-traumatic growth among bereaved people. People with greater authenticity and awareness of life's fragility have heightened existential awareness. Conversely, people who are prone to self-deception and infrequent thoughts of the isolation of existence have less existential awareness.

Although possessing greater existential awareness enhanced people's post-traumatic growth, it didn't alter their grief symptoms or the duration of their bereavement. Drs. Irvin D. Yalom and Morton A. Lieberman, in their 1991 study of heightened existential awareness and bereavement, concluded that examining life deeply after traumatic loss requires the capacity to *look into, rather than away from death, to bear and experience aloneness, to deliberately and willingly face the circumstances of one's life.* Yalom and Lieberman propose that grieving people need internal strength to tolerate loneliness and to candidly appraise their situation. This perspective challenges the notion that grief should be resolved by returning to the way we were before loss; instead, Yalom and Lieberman elevate the power of traumatic loss, where the healthy outcome is self-exploration and personal growth.

The aftermath of loss is a fertile time to see yourself with new eyes—to contemplate how you can compose a life that is fulfilling and realizes your potential. But self-awareness is elusive. Following Bill's death, I searched for the boundary where he ended and I began, and I sensed the tension of differentiating us while also sustaining our bonds. The intermingling of who we were, who he was, and who I had been was like a pile of sand that couldn't be partitioned. At times the blend was unsettling, but it was also a source of comfort. Freud described how ingenious we are at *not knowing* ourselves because of how strictly habit and customs block self-awareness. Routines and social norms allow us to respond automatically rather than thoughtfully and intentionally. So this formative period of loss challenges us to change—to deliberately go down a path where we'll experience emotional pain on the way to becoming more complete.

> But your solitude will be a support and a home for you,
> even in the midst of very unfamiliar circumstances,
> and from it you will find all your paths . . . what we
> call fate does not come into us from the outside, but
> emerges from us.
> —RAINER MARIA RILKE, *Letters to a Young Poet*

Einstein recognized the value of solitude and simplicity in life. *Be a loner,* he said. *That gives you time to wonder, to search for the truth. Have holy curiosity. Make your life worth living.*

Solitude is both a burden and a gift. It's a source of loneliness and the foundation of creativity.

Solitude is the time when our mind wanders; it's when we day-dream. Dr. Kalina Christoff, professor of psychology at the University of British Columbia, who studies the purpose of the wandering mind, describes the presence of *a default brain network* that activates during mind wandering. In both dreaming and mind wandering, the same parts of the brain—the *medial temporal lobes*—are active, sponta-neously generating new thoughts. The brain's control center—*the prefrontal cortex*—then pulls our attention back to purposeful activi-ties. Christoff describes how creativity develops in the interactions between mind wandering and this control center. The control center focuses the mind on issues and problems, while the wandering mind generates creative solutions. But coordination between the control center and mind wandering can be disrupted by anxiety, and creativ-ity is blocked when the amygdala is activated by anxiety and fear. So, relaxation and distraction are essential breaks from the work of confronting loss. Losing yourself in a cherished hobby or favorite TV show, immersing yourself in projects at work, or spending a night out with friends sustains normal routines and recharges our batteries.

There's a fine balance between solitude and socialization. Emo-tional healing is enhanced by being *witnessed*: when our experience is perceived and acknowledged. It's therapeutic to be understood by another human. Humans don't thrive in the absence of relationships; we need eye contact with others, a sense of belonging, and a full range of human interactions, from intimate to casual, from being helped to helping others. Emotional and physical health suffer when we're too isolated. Friends and family are witnesses to our grief and recovery, and counselors may ease us along our way, but some losses may be too intimate to disclose. Words may fail us when we seek to explain our sense of loss to trusted friends. And although counseling is often comforting, we may lack chemistry with a particular therapist.

At times, then, we may find we're our own best witness as we sift through thoughts in our journal and probe the symbols in our dreams. When we pore over the meaning of journal entries—the words we chose, what's said and not said—we bear witness to our own expe-rience. We also bear witness when we examine the odd imagery of our dreams and when we pause to look inward during meditation or prayer. Being witnessed, even by our intimate self, lessens isolation and helps make sense of our situation. By trial and error, we discover the type of witness that brings peace and healing while frequently challenging our own preconceptions.

> Before you eat or drink anything, carefully consider with whom
> you eat or drink rather than what you eat or drink, because
> eating without a friend is the life of the lion or the wolf.
> —EPICURUS, quoted in Daniel Klein's *Travels with Epicurus:*
> *Journey to a Greek Island in Search of a Fulfilled Life*

Fifty years ago, psychiatrists Thomas Holmes and Richard Rahe first published a questionnaire called the Social Readjustment Rating Scale (SSRS), which was designed to measure the social readjustment or stressfulness associated with life events. Thousands of participants rated the amount of life adjustment they needed to handle events from within five categories: death, health, crime, finances, and family. Death of a spouse or partner was associated with the highest stress rating. Other life events with high ratings included the death of close family, a major illness or injury to one's self or one's family, detention in jail, divorce or infidelity, financial difficulties, and being a victim of crime. Social readjustment and stress was also associated with happy occasions, such as marriage, pregnancy, and changes of residence, albeit at lower levels.

Our baseline personality is a key factor in how we handle stressful life experiences. In a 1979 study of stressful life events using the Holmes-Rahe scale, people were divided into groups based on whether they became ill during high stress or remained healthy. Personality analyses showed that the high stress/healthy group had stronger self-esteem and a greater sense of control than the high stress/ill group.

The stress of life experiences is captured by asking survey participants three questions: (1) How unsafe and vulnerable do you feel? (perilousness), (2) Are the stressors unpredictable and random? (unpredictability), and (3) Is the trauma perceived as uncontrollable? (uncontrollability). As psychologists Charles Benight and Albert

Bandura explain, *People live in a psychic environment largely of their own making. To the extent that they can exercise control over what they think, they can regulate how they feel and behave.* If we don't believe our actions will be effective, there's little incentive to persevere in the face of difficulties. This belief in our power to exert control is called *coping self-efficacy*—the term describes our confidence in our ability to handle challenges in the aftermath of traumatic loss. A greater sense of efficacy results in more decisive action, where we act on insights to minimize situations that trigger anxiety and maximize situations that promote clarity and healing. Coping self-efficacy plays a key role in post-traumatic recovery, fostering greater resilience and well-being.

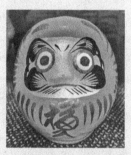

The Daruma is a traditional Japanese doll symbolizing goal setting, resilience, and perseverance. The recipient of the doll paints in one eye (both eyes are initially blank) when setting a goal; they paint the other eye when the goal is fulfilled. Every time the owner sees the one-eyed Daruma, he or she is meant to recall their unrealized goal. When the second eye is finally painted in, the Daruma appears to have both eyes open, symbolizing enlightenment. The Daruma is weighted at the bottom so that it returns to an upright position when tilted, symbolizing resilience.

A Japanese Daruma doll

Our sense of confidence and control stems from many factors, including our personality, resources and support systems, and training and experience. Since life partnerships involve a division of labor, the surviving partner may lack basic knowledge to manage the routine demands of daily living. It's not uncommon for a surviving spouse to lack adequate training to manage household finances (bills, mortgage, insurance), to handle household repairs, or to prepare meals. Even when the fund of knowledge is adequate, managing the estate of the deceased or performing daily activities, such as opening mail addressed to lost loved ones, triggers painful memories. Not knowing—or being able to access—account numbers and passwords further heightens vulnerability and saps confidence.

In their study *I Can, I Do, I Am: The Narrative Differentiation of Self-Efficacy and Other Self-Evaluations while Adapting to Bereavement,* Jack Bauer and George Bonanno explored how people talk during bereavement, differentiating between statements like *I can do things well* (which speaks to self-efficacy), *I do things well* (which speaks to self-management), and *I'm a good person* (which speaks to self-esteem). The hypothesis was that spontaneous expressions of self-efficacy (belief in our ability to do something) is a better predictor of emotional health than statements of self-management or self-esteem. The premise is that redefining personal identity after loss requires personal reflection on not only *what we do*, but also belief in *what we can do* and *can be*. Indeed, speech analysis showed that people *expressing belief in their abilities* had fewer grief symptoms and better adaptation. Statements of belief in what *we can do* reveals our sense of hope and future potential more powerfully than stating *what we're doing*.

The study also found a mental health sweet spot for how we perceive ourselves. Ironically, the best predictor of psychological health is the belief *I'm mostly good, some bad*. In other words, some negative self-evaluation is adaptive, while too little (*I'm not bad*) or too much (*I'm very bad*) is maladaptive—suggesting that balanced self-appraisal leaves room for accepting mistakes and forgiving setbacks. The road to recovery from loss is bumpy—setbacks are frequent and inevitable—so the capacity to accept and be forgiving of our limitations is a key prognostic marker.

The potential for *post-traumatic growth*—or positive change that occurs as a result of struggling with life crises—was first recognized in the mid-90s by psychologists Richard Tedeschi and Lawrence Calhoun. However, not all people experience growth, and some people actually change for the worse after traumatic loss. In a 2004 study, Tedeschi and Calhoun described five types of positive growth: (1) a greater appreciation of life—a changed sense of priorities;

(2) warmer, more intimate relationships with others; (3) a greater sense of personal strength; (4) recognition of new possibilities in life; and (5) spiritual development.

Studies show an unexpected time course for post-traumatic growth. In the *early period* following loss, more post-traumatic growth is seen in people with *greater distress*. In the *intermediate period*, there is no correlation between growth and symptom severity. But then at a *later period*, more post-traumatic growth is seen in people with *less distress*. It appears that early on, greater emotional distress is necessary to trigger and sustain post-traumatic growth. Then over time, sustained growth relieves emotional distress.

In a 1995 study of *the long-term effects* of traumatic loss of a partner or child (two to fifteen years after loss) conducted by Nancy Arbuckle and Brian de Vries, three broad patterns emerged. First, people continued to have lower life satisfaction but greater self-confidence and coping skills; they experienced a combination of negative and positive effects years after the loss. Second, there were gender differences: women tended to have lower self-efficacy (the sense of confidence and control) and to experience greater depression and vulnerability than men. And third, when the impact of education, income, and time since loss were compared, education had the strongest effect of all on function years after loss.

Reflections

When life is interrupted by loss—the breakup of a relationship, the loss of a job, the death of a loved one—there is a time for grief, a time for adaptation, and then an unexpected time of choice and self-determination. It's time to open ourselves up to new possibilities, because the old ones are gone. As time passes, we can't choose if we will age, but we can choose if we will grow. Let's not fail for lack of imagination, determination, or perseverance.

The situation calls for us to employ new strategies to learn about ourselves and leverage our strengths, and to fully open our minds to appraise our situation and interests. *If you were starting all over, what would you do? Where would you live? How would you choose to spend your time? What skills would you seek to develop?* Even when options aren't realistic, it's enlightening to open our minds to take a fresh view. Revise and add to this list over time, considering how new ideas fit in with your present situation and future planning. To get started, make an appraisal of opportunities for *immersion* and *distraction*: time for mindful activities to raise awareness of difficult memories (immersion) and time for rest and rebooting (distraction).

Immersion

- Contemplative practices: journaling, spirituality
- Therapeutic practices: seeing a counselor, joining a support group
- Social interactions focusing on experiences of loss
- Focused learning: reading, classes, lectures

Distraction

- Nature and the outdoors: hiking, biking, birding
- Expressing creativity: drawing, taking photographs, woodworking, writing
- Expanding your horizons: learning new skills
- Lectures, classes, workshops
- Companionship
- Helping others in need
- Organizations: social action, religion, politics, interest groups
- Activity, exercise, recreation
- Old and new hobbies
- Work: bringing fresh energy to old and new projects

Be deliberate and proactive. Avoid continuing activities or remaining in environments that leave you empty or frazzled. Identify things that bring comfort or trigger thoughtful creativity and go after them. Anticipate difficult events before they're upon you, such as holidays and anniversaries. Proactively manage situations that are likely to be challenging. And above all, be patient with and forgiving of yourself—many attempts to attain post-traumatic growth will be unsuccessful. Only by doing will you find out if you're ready for new experiences. If it's too early, or when planning results in missteps, acknowledge your efforts and consider a new path.

> Composing a life involves a continual reimagining of the future and reinterpretation of the past to give meaning to the present, remembering best those events that pre-figured what followed, forgetting those that proved to have no meaning within the narrative. Composing a life involves an openness to possibilities and the capacity to put them together in a way that is structurally sound.
> —MARY CATHERINE BATESON, *Composing a Life*

After five years on my own, it's still a work in progress, but here are things I've learned about myself. I thrive on creativity, personal expression, and challenge. I love to write. Cooking is relaxing, but the kitchen can be a lonely place without Bill by my side. In an over-sharing world, I tend to be private—an obstacle to making human connections. I have strong biorhythms; I'm a dynamo of new ideas in the morning and inevitably subdued in the evening. This translates into optimistic problem-solving as the day begins and pessimistic second thoughts by night.

With new insight, I began to employ those problem-solving skills to daily challenges. To dispel loneliness, I listen to podcasts while cooking and driving; listening to talks on all manner of topics fills the void and prevents rumination. Awakened by demons in the middle of the night, I read book after book by the light of the Kindle; the reading disrupts the mind worms of anxiety and the dim light aids in falling back to sleep. I heed my own biorhythms, shifting to start my day at 5:00 a.m. and establishing a ritual of *immersion*: time for writing between 6:00 and 8:00 a.m. each morning.

But I'm also mindful that adapting to solitude is both an asset and a trap. My greatest challenge stems from how Bill and I built a singular life of devotion to each other. Building a new personal life from scratch continues to be elusive. I've come to recognize the good fortune of being surrounded by family, colleagues, coworkers, patients, students, and neighbors and have newfound respect for opportunities for simple human connection each day. Each step appears so basic, yet the cumulative effect is restorative—less isolation and more sense of purpose.

> The secret to life is finding joy in ordinary things.
> —RUTH REICHL, *My Kitchen Year:*
> *136 Recipes That Saved My Life*

In the second year, I sensed stirrings of something unfamiliar: contentment. It arrived on Mother's Day, a beautiful spring day. Visiting a picturesque garden with family, I took in the colors and fragrance of the flowers and the antics of my grandson romping on the hills and paths. I was able to see, not only watch. I was able to listen, not only hear. I was present in a way I hadn't known since that day three years earlier in Rockport, Maine. I didn't know what was missing until I felt it again: contentment. A sign that life can have value again. Although the path was uncertain, I was stumbling forward.

It's unexpected to find I'm less insecure, stronger. Setbacks have lost much of their sting, cut down to size by confronting a real crisis. I'm more comfortable in my own skin. I'm more present in the moment. Early on, I dwelled on the uncertainty of what will happen; now I'm more patient, trying things out, sowing seeds of potential. I have faith good things will come from the confluence of healing hidden wounds while fostering awareness. At times, I'm caught up in self-doubts, but more often, I believe inner work will transform to direction and purpose. I sense this can't be forced but needs to gestate organically. I acknowledge future possibilities but continue to be realistic about what's been lost: the innocence, the shelter, the joy of the *before life* . . . both a loss and a legacy to build on.

A Pause for Journaling

Describe your personal strengths and weaknesses in developing confidence with managing loss.

In your response, consider these questions:

- Are you independent or dependent?
- Self-revealing or opaque?
- Comfortable being alone or comfortable being with others?

Do you have the knowledge and skills needed to manage your daily activities (finances, meal preparation, household repairs)?

♦

CHAPTER 10

Journaling as a Tool of Emotional Healing

Was it only by dreaming or writing that I could
find out what I thought?
—Joan Didion, *The Year of Magical Thinking*

DOCUMENTING THOUGHTS AND EMOTIONS is hardly a groundbreaking idea, yet the significance of journaling is being reclaimed and connected with the rising interest in mindfulness and well-being. Journaling is creative and therapeutic, with the potential to integrate our conscious and subconscious experience: exactly what's needed during times of emotional trauma and turmoil. Many forms of artistic expression and recreation foster restoration—music, sketching, gardening, yoga—yet journaling uniquely advances self-awareness in one moment while enabling reflection followed by *reflections on reflections* over time. Just as a musician develops greater skill with practice and an athlete develops coordination and strength, the practice of writing down thoughts and feelings develops powers of self-awareness and insight. Creativity has healing powers that awaken and reanimate our emotional life, reconnecting us to the present.

Journaling allows emotional expression without social constraints. Whether we're conversing with friends, family, a counselor, or the members of a support group, what we say and how we say it are constrained by layers of inhibition. Will our words cause alarm? Is this the right time and place to express desolation, loneliness, even hopelessness? Ingrained patterns of behavior often prompt people to offer reflexive assurance to others in order to avoid appearing vulnerable and weak. Expressing raw emotion in private is hard, no less in public settings. In your journal, you can say it any way you want, and you can search for raw truth and authenticity—the antidote for emotional numbness. Journaling fosters insight and self-reliance, while counseling, support groups, and interactions with family and friends tend to foster reliance on others.

Where conversation is in-the-moment, writing is more deliberate, with time to pause and choose words with forethought. Those moments where we hesitate and linger are therapeutic, and they're missing from spoken conversation. As we jot down recollections, momentary thoughts, and descriptions of daily events and inner struggles, the overarching goal is to integrate the experience of loss into our life story, our biography. As images and emotions are transformed into words, they become more organized and coherent. As thoughts and feelings are integrated, subconscious experience begins to surface. Both our memory and what we choose to write in the journal is less random than it appears. There is the initial recollection, the details remembered and those forgotten, and how these memories were molded by time. And then later, we read and relive this experience anew, discovering how old memories connect with new facets of our life. Journaling is a tool to gain access to our experience, to the sensations and thoughts that were present then, and to our interpretation now.

> To write a good memoir you must become the editor
> of your own life, imposing on an untidy sprawl of half-
> remembered events a narrative shape and an organizing
> idea. Memoir is the art of inventing the truth.
> —WILLIAM ZINSSER, *On Writing Well:*
> *The Classic Guide to Writing Nonfiction*

THE SCIENCE OF JOURNALING

James Pennebaker, a psychologist at the University of Texas at Austin, studied how writing about traumatic experience, or *emotionally expressive writing*, results in health benefits, including improved immune, lung, and liver function, reduced blood pressure, fewer doctor visits, and better mood and well-being. Analysis of writing content showed that certain types of writing predicted better adjustment following bereavement, including (1) substantial use of words describing positive emotion, (2) moderate use of words describing negative emotion, and (3) use of words showing insight and causation (realize, understand, reason, because).

Pennebaker's work spurred further studies of the effects of journaling on health outcomes. A review of nine comparable studies showed that journaling produced greater benefits for physical health than mental health among people with diverse medical conditions, including cancer, asthma, rheumatoid arthritis, and PTSD. But not all studies showed benefits: some revealed that people with greater distress (specifically PTSD and prolonged grief) benefited the most from journaling, while other studies indicated that writing about traumatic events actually caused increased emotional distress.

In a study of people with HIV, the virus associated with AIDS, participants assigned to write about emotional topics showed an encouraging drop in viral load and a subsequent rise in CD4 "helper" white blood cell counts. This improvement was not seen in control participants writing about neutral topics. Researchers believe that emotionally expressive writing reduced the participants' stress, which in turn normalized their stress hormone levels and improved their immune function. Next, the study authors wondered, *Is it preferable to express or suppress emotional thoughts?* They assigned participants to write about either emotional or non-emotional topics, with or without suppressing disturbing thoughts. By testing blood drawn before and after writing sessions, the researchers found that both emotional writing *and* thought suppression caused changes in white blood cell counts; these changes indicated the *benefits* of emotional writing and the *detrimental* effects of thought suppression.

In another study, a one-day writing therapy intervention for bereaved family members was conducted. The workshop guided participants to develop a coherent narrative about the death of loved ones and to examine both positive and negative thoughts surrounding this death. The study investigators limited the workshop to a single day to reduce potential negative effects of emotionally expressive writing. When workshop participants were compared to control subjects with no intervention, no differences in outcomes were found. However, there was improvement in the severity of grief symptoms in *all* study participants two months after the study, whether or not they received the intervention. These results show the intrinsic value of time's passage following loss, but doesn't support the hypothesis that writing facilitates healing after loss.

Although the writing intervention failed, there are some important takeaways from this study, as well as a few different ways to interpret the workshop's failure. The simplest and most disheartening explanation is that perhaps writing is simply ineffective. However, comparison with other studies suggests that such a brief writing workshop bypasses the basic healing components of journaling, which include (a) developing insight over time, (b) rereading journal entries to facilitate new insights, and (c) developing an ongoing ritual of mindfulness when pausing to journal. It seems that the time frame and sequence of events is important: in other words, the timing of loss, the duration of expressive writing, and the timing of the assessment of outcomes all contributed to the study's outcome. It's also true that greater self-awareness may result in increased distress at one point, followed by greater emotional comfort later. Writing routines and rituals provide pauses for mindful reflection in the moment and later, for review and reappraisal. Opportunities for discussion of loss with friends and family tend to fade over time, while journaling continues to advance the inner work of adjustment.

Journaling and other meditative practices are potent tools to buffer the *emotional charge* of traumatic loss. Our decision-making and behavior are strongly influenced by this emotional charge. The amygdala, nestled deep in the brain, assigns an emotional weight to events, tagging experiences with their emotional power, their intrinsic positive vs. negative quality, their relative attractiveness or aversiveness. This assigned emotional valence has strong effects on our decisions, actions, and behavior. Judicious decision-making depends upon our capacity to buffer loss's emotional charge; we need personal strategies like journaling to transform the emotional power of loss. As mentioned in earlier chapters, mind wandering and day dreaming are opportunities that spur imagination, opening communication channels between emotions and the mind. As William Zinsser wrote in *On Writing Well*, "Memoir is the art of inventing the truth." To heal the emotional pain of loss, we create new interpretations of our stories, summoning creative energy to plan a new future. In this way, we "try on" different options and envision new possibilities. Loss, whether due to death, divorce, illness, injury, financial instability, or job loss, results in fundamental changes in our daily lives and future plans. We need to use creativity to redefine ourselves and to rethink our identity following loss.

THE "HOW TO" OF JOURNALING

"The only way to compose myself and collect my thoughts,"
he wrote in his diary, "is to set down at my table, place my diary
before me, and take my pen into my hand. This apparatus takes
off my attention from other objects. Pen, ink, and paper and a
sitting posture are great helps to attention and thinking."
—DAVID MCCULLOUGH, *John Adams*

Keeping a journal is simple, particularly since there are no rules: you can do it the way you want, when you want. But there are a few basic guidelines to enhance the personal and restorative qualities of your writing.

1. Be as honest as you can be. It's surprisingly difficult to be fully honest with yourself. You're likely to feel vulnerable and exposed, yet this is how suppressed, unconscious thoughts and feelings will be gradually brought to the surface.

2. Write for yourself and no one else.

3. Keep note paper on hand at all times to record thoughts that come when you least expect them. Be aware of chance encounters and synchronicities that result in new insights.

4. Ignore grammar, form, and style. As Chip Spann writes in *Poet Healer: Contemporary Poems for Health and Healing*, "Keep the pen moving; welcome everything; don't worry about errors; let the subject choose you; write for your eyes only; feelings, feelings, feelings; and details, details, details!"

5. Develop your own writing style. What's your best time of day to write? Do you prefer paper and pencil or computer keyboard? What frequency and duration feel right to you? Whatever style you choose, routine and regularity enhance writing. For example, a daily ritual of easing into a favorite chair first thing in the morning can spark creative expression and clarity of thought. Over time it's as if these cues propel the emotional expression of new ideas and aid in developing your writing style and voice.

6. Always date your journal entries so you can later reflect on evolving themes.

7. Journaling should be reflective and introspective. A journal isn't a calendar; journaling is a tool for discovery and insight.

8. What will you write about? Do you prefer structured or un- structured (open-ended) journaling? Some people believe unstructured journaling results in writing about topics that aren't helpful, or that it results in meaningless rumination. While it's true we may become stuck on certain topics, journaling is a sound strategy to ease us out of the place we're stuck in. The very act of transforming disturbing thoughts that go round and round in our mind into con- crete words, sentences, and paragraphs is an escape valve. We're comforted by seeing these thoughts captured in black and white, where we can return to read them whenever we wish, with no further need to keep them in the forefront of our mind.

My essays begin with "freewriting"—writing without
stopping or self-censorship, free-associative writing.
It is a fertile process that requires me to break through
numbness into desire and memory. That in itself is
reparative and enlarges my self . . . As I move from
freewriting to crafting an essay, I draw on both intellect
and emotion. I am discovering that I love the freedom
of being alone with my ideas and my keyboard.
—JUDITH LINGLE RYAN, *Reweaving the Self:*
Creative Writing in Response to Tragedy

By trial and error, I found an approach that worked for me. With
an erratic schedule of work and travel, establishing a journaling routine was a challenge. I eventually settled on a flexible solution—when
thoughts surface, I jot down notes on small memo pads scattered all
around me: on the bedside table, in my purse, in the car, at my desk.
The results: a few scribbled words while idling at a red light, an illeg-
ible scrawl in the middle of the night, a new insight after soaking in
the tub. These are times when the mind wanders and is receptive to
new insights. When time permits—and my best time is 6:00 a.m.—
I scan the scribbled notes to turn the flurry of disjointed thoughts into
journal entries.

My writing takes many different forms. It may consist of a few
phrases, sentences, or paragraphs, or I may feel moved to expand
the idea into a personal essay. At times I sense these thoughts might
otherwise become distressing ruminations, but focused, expressive
writing disrupts their hold. With time, recollections, thoughts, and
aspirations are woven into a life story, a coherent account of what
happened accompanied by growing self-awareness. It was somewhere
in those first moments of the day, as light crept into the windows,
that the fog began to lift and the sense of being adrift was replaced by
seeds of stability and purpose. No dramatic breakthroughs or epiph-
anies, just a slow process that quietly built over weeks, months, and
years. I simply told and retold those life stories until they began to
make sense to me.

When I write, I am trying through the movement of my
fingers to reach my head. I'm trying to build a word ladder
up to my brain. Eventually these words help me come to
an idea, and then I rewrite and rewrite and rewrite what
I'd already written (when I had no idea what I was writing
about) until the path of thinking, in retrospect, feels
immediate. What's on the page appears to have busted
out of my head and traveled down my arms and through
my fingers and my keyboard and coalesced on the screen.
But it didn't happen like that; it never happens like that.
        —HEIDI JULAVITS, *The Folded Clock: A Diary*

A personal essay expands on memories that linger, suggesting
there's more there than meets the eye. I wrote the following essay
describing a travel experience that, years later, retains many layers
of meaning.

Years ago, I had a colleague who planned and saved for years to
travel to India. As the trip approached his excitement was infectious.
I remember the day I saw him when he returned. He found the trip
disturbing. I always remember that word *disturbing*, because I found
it disturbing. He had seen *disturbing* things he didn't want to talk
about. So years later, when I was invited to give a talk in Mumbai, I
told Bill I planned to decline. Ever the adventurous traveler, Bill was
as persuasive as I was firm. Sensing a serious well of resistance, he
went for a chink in my armor: *You have to go, you're the only woman on
the program.* A few weeks later, we were headed to Mumbai.

A strange, unpleasant smell filled the airplane cabin as we landed
late at night. Surreal: the smog hung heavy in the warm air as we
peered through the car window at faceless bodies sleeping on the
sidewalks. On our arrival at the hotel, the car was surrounded by
men with swords around their waists, wearing fanciful turbans and
colorful costumes adorned with gleaming buttons and braids. They

(continued)

greeted us with great fanfare. We stumbled into our room, falling into deep slumber in that weird space where reality and dreams meet.

India had me from the get-go. Who knew waking up in a strange new world—so surreal it seemed the very laws of science might not apply—could be exhilarating. Sensory overload, sheer chaos to be sure. Cows roamed streets and sidewalks. Monkeys scampered about like oddly aggressive squirrels. There were motor scooters piled high with all manner of wares, even chickens and pigs, weaving through the traffic—other vehicles moved at a snail's pace—and then the occasional elephant or camel would go by. In the country-side, women in jewel-colored saris worked in verdant fields, then walked in a line on the median, large baskets filled with the harvest balanced on their heads. We were surrounded by peddlers beseech-ing us to buy trinkets. A robed man removed the cover of his basket to reveal writhing cobras, and another had a dancing bear on a leash.

One day we took a taxi to the farmers market. As we climbed out of the taxi, the driver said *I'll wait for you.* We assured him, *There's no need.* But leaving the market, we were in a mob, wondering how we'd find a taxi in such chaos. Our taxi driver miraculously appeared— *Here I am*—with a big smile on his face. He eagerly nodded when we told him to drive us back to the hotel, then drove us straight to a carpet shop, where we were surrounded by men bearing trays of refreshing cardamom tea and pastries. *But we want to go back to the hotel,* I kept saying to the driver while Bill dug into the pastries and waved me into the shop. We sat with our refreshments on soft cushions while the silk rugs were rolled out with a thud, then helpers spun each rug around, revealing a hypnotic metamorphosis of color. An enthusiastic collector of everything, Bill was excited by one silk prayer rug and a second with a hunting scene, but not as excited as the salesmen and the taxi driver.

Bill worked his travel magic: our journey took us to New Delhi, Agra (the achingly beautiful Taj Mahal), Khajuraho (temples covered with erotic carvings), Jaipur (the palaces of the great Maharajas), and, most unforgettably, Varanasi, the holiest city of the Hindus.

The devout bring deceased loved ones to Varanasi to be cremated on funeral pyres on the banks of the Ganges. We awakened before dawn and walked in the smoke between the *ghats* (broad stairs descending to the river), then climbed onto a small boat gliding along the river as the sun rose. As the fog receded, we were surrounded by a spectacle of life and death—the glowing pyres, the corpses, the prayerful gatherings of families and priests above, the masses of people bathing in the Ganges below, the echoing sounds of people thrashing clothes against the river stones to cleanse them.

Experiences so extraordinary, so rich, and yes, so disturbing they defy analysis. The days and events washed over us, disrupting preconceptions and unsettling beliefs, as we struggled to take them in. In this way and many others, Bill led me to discover the richness, the texture, the depth of worlds I never knew existed, where travel brings you to a place of new understanding of yourself and the world around you. *Will I ever find this again without him?*

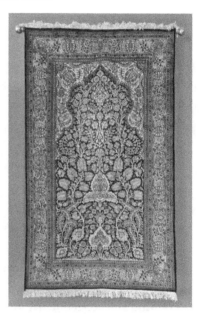

The silk prayer rug from India

What do you want your journal to do for you?

To preserve memories of sacred times.

To tame an onslaught of emotions.

To help you learn from what happened.

To focus the mind and organize your thoughts.

To bring suppressed thoughts out in the open.

To help you reboot, restore, and find balance between internal mindfulness and external connectivity.

> Until you make the unconscious conscious,
> it will direct your life and you will call it fate.
> —CARL JUNG, *The Archetypes*
> *and the Collective Unconscious*

A PAUSE FOR JOURNALING

The following list of questions and themes of loss are starting points or food for thought to pursue in your journal. Impulse is essential to journal writing, but instinct can be balanced by novel ideas and topics.

- If you could change one thing that happened related to your loss, what would it be? Was it something that was under your control? Why or why not?
- When you look back, are there things you did before, during, or after your time of loss that are meaningful to you or satisfying?
- How did you make sense of loss in the moment and how do you interpret the loss now?
- Examine and reflect on activities that bring you a sense of comfort and peace.
- How has loss affected your life story?
- How has loss changed you?
- What are your personal, idiosyncratic interests? Keeping an open mind, think broadly about activities and topics that appeal to you without regard for what seems realistic.
- Loss results in major life changes. What paths are now harder or easier to navigate?

CHAPTER 11

•

Nontraditional and Traditional Therapies
Meditation to Medication

SCIENCE EXPLAINS HOW traumatic loss affects mind and body, but doesn't capture how we feel or the depth of our experience. Following traumatic loss, we're vulnerable and indecisive, not a good starting place to find resources to manage problems: depression, anxiety, isolation, loneliness, sorrow. From the center of this vortex, it's hard to see the big picture, no less summon energy and resources to handle the problem.

Grief is painful. Our reflexive response is avoidance; we try to shut down emotional awareness to avoid suffering. This numbness isn't trivial, since people in need of care are often cut off from therapeutic options. A basic step to raise awareness of our health and well-being is to reconnect with the mind and body by practicing *mindfulness*. The concept of mindfulness has its origins in Buddhism and meditation. Mindful reflection involves focusing attention on present experience with an open, nonjudgmental perspective.

Let's take an open-minded view of what will promote healing during this period. Surely there's no right approach or best approach, as recovery depends on so many things, including individual personality, life experience, the circumstances of loss, and what resources are available. Traditional therapies include counseling, support groups, and antidepressant medications, but options are expanding to include meditation, yoga, cognitive-behavioral therapy, stress management, and structured writing interventions.

Effects of Traditional and Nontraditional Therapies on the Brain

Drugs such as antidepressants have direct effects on the brain, altering both brain chemistry and the messaging between cells in neural pathways. There are many types of antidepressants; using different approaches, they increase the availability of neurotransmitters like serotonin, norepinephrine, and dopamine, thereby strengthening brain pathways that regulate mood. The effects of non-drug holistic therapies on the brain, such as yoga and exercise, are less understood; studies are underway to learn more about them.

Early studies show that meditation causes greater synchronization of brain activity, resulting in positive effects on attention, cognition, and emotion. Antoine Lutz and colleagues from the Department of Psychology at the University of Wisconsin compared brain wave patterns between Buddhists engaged in the practice of meditation for fifteen to forty years to those of control subjects who received meditation training for only one week. The brain wave patterns between the two groups were different at baseline even before an active meditation session. During an active session where both groups focused on a state of unconditional kindness and compassion, the baseline difference in brain wave patterns between the groups sharply increased, showing the long-term effects of routine meditative practice on brain activity.

If regular practice of meditation affects brain activity, does it also affect the brain's physical structure? MRI scans revealed a thicker cerebral cortex in people who regularly practice meditation, particularly in regions of the cortex associated with attention and visual and auditory processing. This suggests that meditation may have the capacity to delay age-related brain atrophy.

Along the same lines, another study investigated the effect of meditation in people with *mild cognitive impairment* (MCI). Half of this group with mild memory problems were trained in mindfulness-based stress reduction, also known as mindfulness meditation; the other half received usual care. On functional MRI, the meditation group showed less atrophy of the hippocampus, a key region for memory function, and increased connectivity between brain regions involved in the default brain network.

Other stress-reducing interventions, such as Tai Chi and aerobic exercise, show similar effects on the brain. Physical exercise has profound brain effects, increasing blood flow to the brain and boosting *nerve growth factors* that enhance neural growth and proliferation. Neural growth involves the lengthening and sprouting of neurons, as well as the development of an enriched network of neural connections. This is precisely what neuroplasticity is: the reorganization of synaptic connections in response to experience or learning. This reorganization is just what people suffering from loss need to promote emotional healing and post-traumatic growth.

Another example of the effects of psychosocial therapy on the brain comes from a clinical trial investigating the effectiveness of *stress-management therapy* (SMT) to prevent new brain lesions in the neurologic disorder multiple sclerosis (MS). When MS patients receiving SMT were compared to a control group (MS patients who were not receiving SMT), brain imaging showed less active disease in the MS patients receiving the stress-management therapy: in other words, fewer MS lesions and less brain atrophy. Although these studies were not performed on people experiencing traumatic loss, they show consistent effects of meditation and other psychosocial therapies on the structure and function of the brain and demonstrate how non-pharmacologic therapies can make a difference.

Psychosocial and Holistic Therapies

People respond differently to traumatic loss. Because their symptoms vary, it's essential to understand if the main problem is grief, or whether there are additional components of depression or anxiety. They may also be suffering from other problems that need to be addressed, such as insomnia or panic attacks. The difference between depression and grief may not be obvious. Basic definitions describe depression as *sadness with diminished interest in things*, while grief is defined as *deep sorrow and suffering* related to a loss. One might say that depression makes us feel hollow—it's an absence of joy, while grief is active and tormenting. Anxiety is also distinct: it involves a sense of unease and fearfulness. Although the experiences of depression, anxiety, and grief are all different, they commonly occur together. The main point is that remedies should be selected based on the symptoms of concern; one size doesn't fit all. Studies show that counseling is helpful in treating people for depression and anxiety, but less effective for people suffering from symptoms of grief, whether related to trauma, loss, or bereavement. These results are prompting development of many new and innovative approaches for grief symptoms.

For example, novel models of psychotherapy targeted toward people experiencing more intense symptoms of prolonged grief are showing promising results. Cognitive-behavioral therapy (CBT) programs developed for complicated grief are more structured and devote more time to deliberate exposure to the loss experience than general counseling. CBT may include diverse components, including cognitive restructuring, reflective writing, psychoeducation, and emotional regulation training. Overall, accumulating evidence shows that *avoidance* of reminders of loss doesn't reduce emotional distress or promote post-traumatic growth in the long term. On the contrary, exposure to painful emotions and memories is a difficult but necessary step on the path of healing.

What type of therapy will work best for you? Baseline personality traits may predict whether group therapy will be successful or not. The most favorable outcomes in group therapy are seen in people who tend to be more talkative and optimistic (extroverted), as well as more organized and disciplined (conscientious). Being intellectually curious and comfortable with new experience also favors success in therapy (openness).

This makes quite a bit of sense. If you're extroverted, your sociable nature fosters enthusiasm for participating in therapy. When you're conscientious, you tend to work harder in therapy and tolerate emotional discomfort for later rewards. Conversely, the predisposition to be more anxious and depressed tends to result in poor adaptation, more self-consciousness, and less favorable outcomes in therapy.

In 1997, H. A. W. Schut and colleagues investigated gender differences in response to therapy for bereavement by comparing the effects of two different types of counseling: problem-focused vs. emotion-focused programs. A compelling hypothesis based on conventional wisdom was that women would benefit more from the emotion-focused intervention, while the men would do better with the problem-focused approach, but the results showed just the opposite!

Conventional wisdom suggested that women and men would do best with interventions that supplemented or boosted their usual coping strategies. However, although women tend to use emotion-based strategies, they received greater benefit when they were counseled using a problem-focused approach. The men were in the reverse situation: although they tend to use problem-focused strategies, they received more benefit from emotion-based counseling.

The take-home message: these results support novel and challenging approaches over reliance on customary coping strategies. We're likely to receive greater benefit by adding new strategies to our arsenal.

Increasingly, novel and innovative approaches to bereavement are being introduced. Internet-based programs, shown to be effective for anxiety and depression, are now available for people suffering from symptoms of loss, grief, and trauma. A comparison of therapist-guided, internet *exposure therapy* versus *behavioral activation* showed improved grief symptoms and reduced post-traumatic stress with both approaches. *Exposure therapy* gradually exposes individuals to difficult memories associated with loss to reduce avoidance. *Behavioral activation* therapy fosters gradual engagement in meaningful and fulfilling activities. Physical activity (stationary bicycle and other aerobic exercise), resistance training, and yoga were studied as treatment for post-traumatic stress disorder and found to reduce PTSD and depressive symptoms. Physical training is likely to have added advantages for physical health and sleep.

Eastern philosophies and holistic health practices open new avenues to manage grief and loss. Key components include (a) developing trust in our inner strength, (b) accepting life's dynamic state and its search for equilibrium, (c) gaining confidence in our ability to turn crises into transformative opportunities for growth, and (d) believing that small changes can result in new synergies of well-being. Varied techniques, including massage, yoga, Tai Chi, storytelling, and physical exercise, may all contribute to spiritual integrity. In "East meets West: Applying Eastern Spirituality in Clinical Practice," Cecilia Chan and colleagues describe how Eastern spirituality aides us in finding a middle path between battling adversity and giving in by both fighting for change and accepting fate.

Psychosocial interventions reduce emotional distress, but do they also foster post-traumatic growth? Rising interest in post-traumatic growth is spurring new programs that explicitly aim to promote stress-related growth and find meaning after adversity. These programs include many of the CBT components previously described, with greater emphasis on meaning-making, gaining wisdom, developing narratives that foster post-traumatic growth, and exploring new life principles. Early evidence shows that focused interventions promote psychological and emotional growth following traumatic loss.

When mindfulness exercises in a bereavement support group were studied by Michael Kogler and colleagues, two types of benefit were found: these exercises fostered (1) social support (a sense of belonging and help from others) and (2) self-regulation (better acceptance of loss and orientation toward the future). Many people are aided by support groups, but my own experience was disappointing. Discussion was tangential; a bounty of opportunities to kindle the inner work of grieving were passed over. The facilitator was hesitant to broach upsetting topics or to suggest that life can have meaning after loss. Although I recognized this wasn't working out, that I needed new options, I floundered. Keep in mind that not all attempts to find support will be successful; each of us knows when we connect with a genuine, meaningful approach.

Spirituality and Religion

Albert Einstein waded into the difficult terrain at the interface of science and religion. One month before Einstein died, he learned a close colleague had passed away. In a letter of condolence, he wrote, *He has departed from this strange world a little ahead of me. That means nothing. For us believing physicists, the distinction between past, present and future is only a stubborn illusion.*

> The most beautiful emotion we can experience is the mysterious. It is the fundamental emotion that stands at the cradle of all true art and science . . . To sense that behind anything that can be experienced there is something that our minds cannot grasp, whose beauty and sublimity reaches us only indirectly: this is religiousness. In this sense, and in this sense only, I am a devoutly religious man.
>
> —ALBERT EINSTEIN, quoted in Walter
> Isaacson's *Einstein: His Life and Universe*

Einstein concluded with the famous quote, *Science without religion is lame, religion without science is blind.* This is relevant to the profound experience of loss and our exploration of how science explains experience and promotes healing. Religion, spirituality, and science can coexist—our experience is greater than the sum of its parts. For some, religion is a deep source of support and emotional restoration, while others find comfort from diverse spiritual practices. Still others feel estranged from religion as they ask how God allows suffering. *Why did God let this happen?*

Wherever we fit on this spectrum, the experience of traumatic loss spurs existential thoughts with spiritual and religious connotations. Loss is often accompanied by rituals that may have intense religious meaning, or may simply mark a moment in time as worthy of attention and respect. In an earlier chapter, I described the rabbi's visit with Bill on his last day. In this harrowing time, the recitation of the Viddui, a prayer spoken when death is imminent, was the single most meaningful event. This ancient ritual filled an intense need for both of us. A religious or spiritual tradition can be a vital pathway to deep emotions. *Subconscious-Conscious Integration*, previously described as a key principle, requires a *pathway in*. Our inner nature determines what traumatic memories are suppressed and inaccessible; these are the experiences that touched us the most and that need to be surfaced again. Religion and spirituality, in their many forms, are important tools that help us find a pathway in, unearthing hidden emotions and memories.

> I have always been able to pray for the other dead, and I still do, with some confidence. But when I try to pray for H., I halt. Bewilderment and amazement come over me. I have a ghastly sense of unreality, of speaking into a vacuum about a nonentity. The reason for the difference is only too plain. You never know how much you really believe anything until its truth or falsehood becomes a matter of life and death to you . . . Apparently the faith—I thought it faith—which enables me to pray for the other dead has seemed strong only because I never really cared, not desperately, whether they existed or not. Yet I thought I did.
>
> —C. S. LEWIS, *A Grief Observed*

In his essay "Ascending the Spiral Staircase of Grief," Sameet Kumar describes three "pearls of understanding" to aid in *transforming the suffering of grief into a meaningful life transition*. The first pearl: *Grief is often nonlinear*. Kumar compares the path of grief to a spiral staircase—a natural cycle that ebbs and flows with an overall trajectory of rising growth. The second pearl: *Normalize the universality of death in the human experience to facilitate acceptance of grief*. Grief is intimate and isolating. The recognition that witnessing death is a universal experience dispels isolation and recalls the community of people around us who confront the same challenges. Buddhism describes the journey to spiritual maturity as opening to what life presents rather than resisting—letting life be as it is rather than demanding it conform to our wishes. The third pearl: *Mindfulness is a transformative technique for facilitating meaning-making in times of grief and identity transition. In times of great loss, most of us find that our identities consist primarily of the relationships we have.* When our identity is challenged by loss, we struggle to reestablish balance and stability. Finding channels and opportunities for mindfulness are essential for introspection, self-care, and new decisions.

DRUG THERAPIES

Antidepressant medications are often used to treat symptoms of grief, but are they effective? Studies of antidepressant medications show these drugs are more effective for treating symptoms of depression than symptoms of grief. No single antidepressant is better than others: a variety of antidepressant medications have been shown to be both effective and safe, including buproprion (Wellbutrin), escitalopram (Lexapro), nortriptyline (Pamelor), paroxetine (Paxil), and sertraline (Zoloft).

Charles F. Reynolds, geriatric psychiatrist at the University of Pittsburgh, compared four different approaches to treating bereavement-related depression: (1) antidepressant therapy alone (nortriptyline), (2) antidepressant therapy plus psychotherapy, (3) a placebo alone, and (4) a placebo plus psychotherapy. The four treatments clearly differed in their effects on depressive symptoms, with the greatest effect seen in those receiving both antidepressants and psychotherapy (69% of the group improved). The smallest effect on depression was in the group receiving a placebo plus psychotherapy; only 29% improved. Antidepressants alone resulted in a 56% improvement, and a placebo alone resulted in a 45% improvement, demonstrating the power of the placebo effect. Although depression improved to some degree with all four approaches, there was no difference between the four groups in terms of a lessening of grief intensity. In less reliable studies of antidepressant effects that lack a control (placebo) group, depressive symptoms improved in 50 to 70% of all study subjects, while grief symptoms improved in 5 to 50% of the subjects. Overall, studies of antidepressant medications show that medications may be more effective than counseling for depression, but not for symptoms of grief.

TAKEAWAY MESSAGES ABOUT MANAGEMENT

Putting this all together, sound evidence supports the effectiveness of a broad range of approaches to improve symptoms after traumatic loss. Key takeaway messages are: (1) depressive symptoms and grief symptoms are distinct—they respond differently to treatment; and (2) medications and psychosocial interventions have different effects. Medications are effective for treating depression and anxiety, but are not likely to directly reduce the intensity of grief. Psychosocial interventions may be effective for treating depression and anxiety and may also improve symptoms of grief. Paradoxically, grief symptoms respond best when they're more intense and prolonged: the vulnerable subgroup of people with greater grief severity benefits the most from treatment and these gains are more easily measured. But this vulnerable subgroup is also at the greatest risk of remaining invisible to supportive services despite the fact that they desperately need attention.

A limitation of scientific studies is that they're generally better at evaluating distinct interventions than seeing the big picture—the sum of the parts. For example, common symptoms of depression (hopelessness, fatigue, loss of motivation) are likely to interfere with efforts to initiate and sustain common treatment approaches, like attending an exercise class or support group. Social interaction at a support group may spark ideas in grieving people, leading to new resources and options. From this perspective, the most effective strategy for promoting recovery is likely to involve combining diverse approaches.

Some of the approaches described in this chapter may appear unfamiliar—however, that also describes the place we find ourselves after traumatic loss. The ambiguity of grief is a gateway, a time to suspend disbelief and open ourselves to new approaches and possibilities: to experiment with meditation and yoga, to try one's hand at expressive writing, or to reengage in religious ritual. Thinking back to the approach that Bill and I adopted after his diagnosis, uncertainty calls for behaving *as if*. Without the certainty of knowing what will work or won't work, we can freely explore what will help us climb back on solid ground. When experimenting with new options, practice precedes confidence and commitment. Going through the motions of new routines gradually acquires deeper and deeper meaning.

A Pause for Journaling

This chapter describes a range of nontraditional and traditional approaches to alleviate symptoms associated with loss. Approaches include counseling, psychotherapy, support groups, meditation, antidepressant medications, yoga, Tai Chi, physical exercise, stress-management training, structured writing interventions, and spiritual or religious practices.
In this context, make an appraisal of your experience.

- What have you tried and not tried?
- What has or has not been helpful?
- Describe your impression of the options. Reviewing each option, which seems (a) promising, (b) unfamiliar, but may have possibilities, or (c) not your thing?
- Is your personality or past experience a guide to what approaches are likely to be most effective for you?
- Now consider less familiar, more daring, options. What's on this list?

CHAPTER 12

•

Emotional Restoration

A Gateway to New Directions

We'd board the plane and toast the start of each journey. Over glasses of champagne, Bill told the story of what he'd planned. Not much detail; just enough to whet the appetite and let my mind roam over the broad outlines of the coming adventure. Each day, he conceived the reveal, composing journeys that defined us. On a whisky tour in Scotland, we drove through chilly drizzle, visited seaside inns, savored whisky oatmeal to dispel the morning chill, and sipped scotch as the sun set over the Bay of Oban. The next day, a ferry to the island of Iona—we hiked to the Abbey and admired the ancient Celtic cross. One morning, Bill drove for hours, destination unknown, passing countless sheep. A picturesque cottage came into view, where the receptionist awaited us with a romantic lunch by the fire.

MEMORIES BURNISHED TO A FINE PATINA. Memories like a swirl of colors in a can of paint, colors of longing mixed with colors of warmth and grace. But now, there's no loss of time or awareness; the world doesn't vanish. I focus, I reflect, I remember. The time has come to find my center and create a fresh path.

When are you going to get on with your life?

The question is unsettling, judgmental, disorienting.

People ask this with concern (*it's unhealthy*), with reproach (*it's unwanted*), with impatience (*it's unseemly*).

The implication is that my time course isn't meeting expectations.

Or life should return to what it was.

Or it's not healthy to dwell on the past.

They say, *It's time to get on with your life.*

There's something here that captures the experience after loss, the gap between experience and expectations, the disconnect between our choices and popular assumptions.

The choices are many. Some find comfort with friends and family, while others immerse themselves in work and activity. Some take a break or hiatus, and others feel the urge to sell their home or move to a new city. After losing a life partner, some are driven to find a new partner, while others build a new life alone.

Grief is individual and personal—*the depth of grief reflects the depth of loss.* Common expectations of behavior after loss fail to acknowledge individual experience. There are so many paths to follow—do they all lead to healing, restoration, and growth? *Do all roads lead to the same place?* Healing comes with time, but post-traumatic growth comes from insight and awareness.

The capacity for self-determination is based on insight and instinct, an awareness of where we've been and where we're going. Uncertainty about the future is uncomfortable, unnerving, even harrowing. It's difficult to get in touch with what we want for ourselves, what brings genuine satisfaction and meaning to our lives. It's less complicated to make choices that avoid uncertainty than to choose the longer road of inner work and personal insight.

> Sometimes I feel removed from my peers because I
> feel less concern about minor passing events and styles.
> However, I can accept that because I feel I do have a
> firm grip on what is and is not of importance. I think
> I will have to learn to deal with the strain about doing

the things that will enrich my life instead of the things
society may expect of me.

—IRVIN D. YALOM, *Staring at the Sun:*
Overcoming the Terror of Death

Science shows the neurologic correlates of emotional symptoms.
As knowledge of the neurology of grief expands, conventional wisdom
on the experience of loss and emotional trauma trails behind. The
manifestations of grief, from depression to hopelessness, from dissociative symptoms to emotional pain, are evidence of altered brain
function. We no longer view depression after stroke or in Parkinson's
or Alzheimer's disease as expected emotional consequences of living
with a medical condition; depression, we understand, is as much a
symptom of the underlying brain disorder as paralysis, tremor, or de-
mentia. Similarly, grief is a manifestation of neurologic trauma, and
is evidence of injury to brain regions that regulate emotions.

Grieving is a healthy, protective process. It's an evolutionary adap-
tation to promote survival in the face of emotional trauma, one where
the injury goes undetected since daily function is preserved.

Our brain's neural pathways are remodeled in response to experience, both good and bad. This is precisely what neuroplasticity is:
the reorganization of synaptic connections in response to experience
or learning. So neuroplasticity moves in both directions, changing in
response to traumatic loss, and then changing again in response to restorative experience. The brain's limbic system is on heightened alert
after traumatic stress, but *neurons trained to be on overdrive can be*
tamed by periods of meditation and warm companionship. And as the
brain's neurons and neurochemistry change, our emotional experience
and behavior changes. Neuroplasticity is needed for emotional healing
and post-traumatic growth. This step-by-step process moves us from
that disquieting sense of instability to regaining equilibrium.

As these chapters slowly took form, the experience of loss became
part of my life story—something concrete that makes sense to me.
I now understand not only what happened, but how it altered the
function of mind and brain, and in that process changed me. Only we

can do this inner work; no one can do it for us; there's no simple path and no shortcut.

I am in mortal danger.

When I broke the silence with these words in Bill's final days, they came from a place beneath awareness, revealing a split between my conscious and subconscious where the conscious mind wasn't ready for this message and the subconscious was imperiled. But there was no sudden breakthrough of insight that day, or on any day to follow. All remained buried and hidden, waiting to be slowly uncovered layer by layer.

During an office visit with a person with Parkinson's, I asked how he's handling disability, specifically the increasing slowness and loss of dexterity of his fingers and hands. *You know, Dr. Shulman, it feels like just the right pace to me . . . you need to reset your goals.* His words remind us how the quality of our lives is determined by how we interpret our experiences, not by the experiences. The aftermath of emotional trauma isn't recovery, it's restoration. We aren't healed, we're different; some things are lost and some are gained. We may lose optimism and innocence but we gain maturity, insight, and empathy. *You need to reset your goals.*

This book isn't about Bill and me; our story is simply the proxy of many stories where tenacious bonds are ripped apart by traumatic events and severed attachments continue to search for their natural connections. These bonds are etched in the fiber of our being, imprinted in our neural circuitry, and result in foreseeable symptoms of grief, sometimes mistaken for anomaly, by both the sufferer and observer. But as these severed attachments scar and heal, new shoots appear and grow, giving way to new growth possessed of wisdom of what was.

A part of me continues to look at the world through Bill's eyes, to be moved by things that moved him. On a lunch date at Bill's favorite Russian restaurant, I order the dishes he loved: a shot of chilled coriander vodka, a plate of herring with dark bread, a fresh beet salad. People say those we lose live on inside us. Before, a cliché—but after, there it is.

I still reflect on things I don't fully understand about those times: our inability to speak frankly about Bill's approaching death and what he envisioned for my future. He never said. I think it goes back to who he was and who we were together. He didn't analyze, he was instinctive. He accepted life's difficulties, sustaining the conviction that *Things will go well*, with no sense of contradiction. He was comfortable in his skin and comfortable with ambiguity. And I love these parts of his nature—his legacy.

These chapters trace a long path that follows my instinct that healing will grow from understanding. As I returned to read and reread my own words, I found meaning in the written word, in the unwritten word, and in the space between the words. How do we move forward after loss? How do we honor our past and grow, and not be diminished by emotional trauma? In these chapters, the sequence of events and insights unfolds in a neat package, as if events were comprehensible in real time. Quite the opposite: the events were amplified by time to crystallize insight. Early on, I sensed something odd was happening— that altered state of mind—and I went searching for answers.

The process of emotional healing and brain healing is enhanced by a balance of activities and experiences, some distracting and some challenging, some physical and some emotional, some social and some private. All the while, we are searching for a fine balance, a balance that tips back and forth from restful to jarring, from camaraderie to overstimulation, from meditation to isolation. *Try a lot of things to figure this out.* Summon energy to try new things: join a gym or yoga class or follow a creative urge in drawing or photography. Be open to the healing powers of the outdoors. Take on a new challenge at work. Plan a travel adventure. Volunteer in your community, church, or temple. Become a docent in the local museum or pitch in during a political campaign. Assemble reading and movie lists; return to those classics you missed. Intersperse things you enjoy with content that focuses on loss, making time to reflect on your experience while contemplating the experience of others. Then dive into something completely diverting to cleanse and refresh the mind. This aligns with the three principles I described in chapter 5: Employing *Immersion–*

Distraction to promote *Subconscious–Conscious Integration* and to lay the groundwork for *Opening the Mind to Possibilities.*

---◆---

FOUR YEARS SINCE BILL'S DEATH

I'm in an airport leaving for vacation, when I realize I've lost my suitcase. I retrace my steps but can't find it. To report the loss, I complete a questionnaire—but I can't recall what city I'm in or where I'm going. I try to sound normal while asking the clerk, *What city are we in?* Now I can't find my ticket and I miss my flight.

COMMENT: *Four years later, it's still a work in progress. Daily life is filled with purpose and my emotional life is steady. These "journey dreams" filled with disorganization and disorientation are less frequent, but not gone—a persistent echo of the ambiguity of the future.*

---◆---

Somewhere along this road, we learn more about ourselves—our strengths and weaknesses, our personal preferences, our aspirations and dreams. With time and space for reflection, we search for answers. Whatever time we have left, how do we want to spend it? With hard-earned wisdom, what is genuine and meaningful? In this fast-paced, accelerating world, loss is a turning point, a time to ponder personal goals, to thoughtfully compose *our after life.* If we're going to make radical changes—move to a new city, find a new home, leave the workplace—let it be with the diligence big decisions demand. Let's not run away from a burning building, let's calmly walk the well-chosen path.

> It is perfectly true, as the philosophers say, that life must be understood backwards. But they forget the other proposition, that it must be lived forwards.
> —SØREN KIERKEGAARD

Acknowledgments

Many people—family, friends, colleagues, advisors, doctors, nurses—
are integral to these events.

Bill's loss endures for many, especially Miriam and Monica Weiner,
Gregg Bellows, Abel and Adam Bellows, Barry and Linda Weiner, and
Merle Weiner and Art Goldberg. The impact of these events continues
for Josh, Esther, Emily, and Julie Shulman, and Corey, Jenna, Micah,
and Brett Shulman. I'm grateful for the support and encouragement
from all and many others: Mitchell Mink, Jackie Gilson, Arthur and
Marcia Stamberg, Edith Gering, and Shelly and Sue Gering.

There were combined personal and professional losses for many
friends and colleagues at the University of Maryland Department of
Neurology, including Stephen Reich, Paul Fishman, Alan and Fran-
cine Krumholz, Bryan and Diane Soronson, Howard Eisenberg, and
especially Barney Stern, who has traveled a similar path. Bill and I
are indebted to our administrative and nursing staff, including Cheryl
Grant-Johnson, Cherika Jones, Nancy Zappala, and Michelle Cines,
who managed the repercussions of Bill's illness on our research and
departmental operations. I want to honor the memory of the former
chair of neurology, Dr. Kenneth Johnson, and to recognize the kindness and support of the dean of the University of Maryland School of
Medicine, Dr. Albert Reese.

Difficult times during Bill's illness were eased by contact with
close friends, especially Stewart Factor and Steven Ringel. I want to
thank Basil Anderman for his sage advice during the early weeks of
mourning. Colleagues and friends at the American Academy of Neurology and the American Brain Foundation are too numerous to list.
During difficult times, they were an island of stability in a world that
was tilting.

Doctors and nurses carry an added burden when caring for a colleague. I'm grateful for the expertise and humanity of Bill's physicians,

Dr. Robb Stein in Rockport, Maine, and Drs. Ashraf Badros, Young Kwok, and Kevin Cullen at the University of Maryland Greenebaum Cancer Center. I recognize the skill and compassion of the nurses caring for Bill in the Stoler Infusion Center, led by Todd Milliron.

Our patients are an enduring source of support and inspiration— for Bill during his illness, and for me during difficult times.

Johns Hopkins University Press encouraged me to keep going, which is not at all trivial. Many thanks for editorial expertise and guidance from Joe Rusko, Jackie Wehmueller, Hilary Jacqmin, Jane Sapal, and Greg Britton. The cited references are a tiny sample of the hundreds of publications uncovered by Andrea Shipper at the University of Maryland Health Sciences Library. Finally, I'm grateful for editorial advice from Joan Blumberg, Mitchell Waters, and Michael Ballard.

As the book recounts, Rabbi Daniel Burg brought dignity and meaning to Bill's final days. Reverend Walter Smith's advice and experience with bereavement was fundamental to sharpening the focus of my work on grief from the perspective of a neurologist.

Inevitably, people have been overlooked—your contributions are no less important. The words that appear between these covers were shaped by many exceptional people who influenced our lives.

Bibliography

Chapter 1. But We Will

Figure on page 5: Pierre-Auguste Renoir, French, 1841–1919. *Dance at Bougival*, 1883. Oil on canvas. 181.9 × 98.1 cm (71⅝ × 38⅝ in.). Museum of Fine Arts, Boston. Picture Fund. 37.375.

Yalom ID. *Staring at the Sun: Overcoming the Terror of Death*. San Francisco, CA: Jossey-Bass; 2009.

Chapter 3. We Are Dying

Bateson MC. *With a Daughter's Eye: A Memoir of Margaret Mead and Gregory Bateson*. New York: HarperCollins; 1984.

Tolstoy L. *The Death of Ivan Ilyich*. MA: Seven Treasures Publications; 2009.

Chapter 4. The Altered Life

de Vries B, Utz R, Caserta M, Lund D. Friend and family contact and support in early widowhood. *Journals of Gerontology. Series B: Psychological Sciences and Social Sciences*. 2014;69(1):75–84.

Kahneman D, Slovic P, Tversky A. *Judgment Under Uncertainty: Heuristics and Biases*. New York: Cambridge University Press; 1982.

Khayyám O. *The Rubáiyát of Omar Khayyám*. FitzGerald E., trans. New York: Garden City Publishing; 1917.

Lewis CS. *A Grief Observed*. New York: HarperCollins; 1994. First published 1961 by N.W. Clerk.

Penman EL, Breen LJ, Hewitt LY, Prigerson HG. Public attitudes about normal and pathological grief. *Death Studies*. 2014;38:8:510–516.

Tippett K. *Becoming Wise: An Inquiry into the Mystery and Art of Living*. New York: Penguin Press; 2016.

Chapter 5. The Neurology of Grief

Bonanno GA, Keltner D, Holen A, Horowitz MJ. When avoiding unpleasant emotions might not be such a bad thing: Verbal-autonomic response dissociation and midlife conjugal bereavement. *Journal of Personality and Social Psychology*. 1995;69(5):975–989.

Bui E, Simon NM, Robinaugh DJ, Leblanc NJ, Wang Y, Skritskaya NA, et al. Periloss dissociation, symptom severity, and treatment response in complicated grief. *Depression and Anxiety*. 2013;30:123–128.

Didion J. *The Year of Magical Thinking.* New York: Alfred Knopf; 2006.

Greenspan D. *Around My French Table: More than 300 Recipes from My Home to Yours.* Boston: Houghton Mifflin Harcourt; 2010.

Karjala LM. *Understanding Trauma and Dissociation: A Guide for Therapists, Patients and Loved Ones.* Atlanta: ThomasMax Publishing; 2007.

Lewis CS. *A Grief Observed.* New York: HarperCollins; 1994. First published 1961 by N.W. Clerk.

Yalom ID. *Creatures of a Day and Other Tales of Psychotherapy.* New York: Basic Books; 2015.

Chapter 6. Dreams and Dream Interpretation

Belicki K, Gulko N, Ruzycki K, Aristotle J. Sixteen years of dreams following spousal bereavement. *OMEGA - Journal of Death and Dying.* 2003; 47(2):93–106.

Boa F. *The Way of the Dream: Conversations on Jungian Dream Interpretations with Marie-Louise von Franz.* Boston: Shambhala; 1994.

Edwards CL, Ruby PM, Malinowski JE, Bennett PD, Blagrove MT. Dreaming and insight. *Frontiers in Psychology.* 2013;4(979):1–14.

Fox KCR, Nijeboer S, Solomonova E, Domhoff GW, Christoff K. Dreaming as mind wandering: Evidence from functional neuroimaging and first-person content reports. *Frontiers in Human Neuroscience.* 2013;7(412):1–18.

Freud S, Strachey J. *The Interpretation of Dreams: The Complete and Definitive Text.* Philadelphia: Basic Books; 2010.

Hobson JA. *Consciousness.* New York: W. H. Freeman; 1999.

Landmann N, Kuhn M, Maier JG, Spiegelhalder K, Baglioni C, Frase L, et al. REM sleep and memory reorganization: Potential relevance for psychiatry and psychotherapy. *Neurobiology of Learning and Memory.* 2015;122:28–40.

Von Unwerth M. *Freud's Requiem: Mourning, Memory, and the Invisible History of a Summer Walk.* New York: Riverhead Books; 2005.

Wagner U, Gais S, Heider H, Verleger R, Born J. Sleep inspires insight. *Nature.* 2004;427:352–355.

Walker MP, Liston C, Hobson JA, Stickgold R. Cognitive flexibility across the sleep-wake cycle: REM-sleep enhancement of anagram problem solving. *Cognitive Brain Research.* 2002:14(3):317–324.

Williams KL. Dreams of life and death. *Psychological Perspectives.* 2015;58(1): 34–43.

Worden JW. *Grief Counseling and Grief Therapy: A Handbook for the Mental Health Practitioner.* 4th ed. New York: Springer Publishing; 2008.

Wright ST, Kerr CW, Doroszczuk NM, Kuszczak, Hang PC, Luczkiewicz KL. The impact of dreams of the deceased on bereavement: A survey of hospice caregivers. *American Journal of Hospice and Palliative Medicine.* 2014;31(2):132–138.

Chapter 7. The Science of the Wounded Mind

For more about categories of risk factors discussed on page 87, see full citations below for Bangasser and Valentino, "Sex differences"; Breen and O'Connor, "Fundamental paradox"; Logue et al., "Psychiatric genomics consortium."

American Psychiatric Association. *Diagnostic and Statistical Manual of Mental Disorders, DSM–5*, 5th ed. Washington, DC: American Psychiatric Publishing, 2013.

Arbuckle NW, de Vries B. The long-term effects of later life spousal and parental bereavement on personal functioning. *The Gerontologist*. 1995;35(5):637–647.

Assareh AA, Sharpley CF, McFarlane JR, Sachdev PS. Biological determinants of depression following bereavement. *Neuroscience and Biobehavioral Reviews*. 2015;49:171–181.

Bangasser DA, Valentino RJ. Sex differences in stress-related psychiatric disorders: Neurobiological perspectives. *Frontiers in Neuroendocrinology*. 2014;35:303–319.

Breen LJ, O'Connor M. The fundamental paradox in the grief literature: A critical reflection. *OMEGA - Journal of Death and Dying*. 2007;55(3):199–218.

Freud S. *Mourning and Melancholia*. In: Strachey J, trans-ed. *The Standard Edition of the Complete Psychological Works of Sigmund Freud*. Vol. 14, 1917. Reprint, London Hogarth Press; 1957.

Galatzer-Levy IR, Bryant RA. 636,120 ways to have posttraumatic stress disorder. *Perspectives on Psychological Science*. 2013;8(6):651–662.

Gilbertson MW, Shenton ME, Ciszewski A, Kasai K, Lasko NB, Orr SB, et al. Smaller hippocampal volume predicts pathologic vulnerability to psychological trauma. *Nature Neuroscience*. 2002;5:1242–1247.

Gundel H, O'Connor MF, Littrell L, Fort C, Lane RD. Functional neuroanatomy of grief: An fMRI study. *American Journal of Psychiatry*. 2003;160:1946–1953.

Kelley LP, Weathers FW, McDevitt-Murphy ME, Eakin DE, Flood AM. A comparison of PTSD symptom patterns in three types of civilian trauma. *Journal of Traumatic Stress*. 2009;22(3):227–235.

Logue MW, Amstadter AB, Baker DG, Duncan L, Koenan KC, Liberzon I, et al. The psychiatric genomics consortium posttraumatic stress disorder workgroup: Posttraumatic stress disorder enters the age of large-scale genomic collaboration. *Neuropsychopharmacology*. 2015;40:2287–2297.

Mancini AD, Bonanno GA. Resilience in the face of potential trauma: Clinical practices and illustrations. *Journal of Clinical Psychology: In Session*. 2006;62:971–985.

Miller MD. Complicated grief in later life. *Dialogues in Clinical Neuroscience*. 2012;14(2):195–202.

Murray JA. Loss as a universal concept: A review of the literature to identify common aspects of loss in diverse situations. *Journal of Loss and Trauma*. 2001;6(3):219–241.

O'Connor MF. Bereavement and the brain: Invitation to a conversation between bereavement researchers and neuroscientists. *Death Studies.* 2005;29:905–922.

Parkes CM, Weiss RS. *Recovery from Bereavement.* New York: Basic Books; 1983.

Rutten BPF, Hammels C, Geschwind N, Menne-Lothmann C, Pishva E, Schruers K, et al. Resilience in mental health: Linking psychological and neurobiological perspectives. *Acta Psychiatrica Scandinavica.* 2013;128:3–20.

Shear MK. Complicated grief. *New England Journal of Medicine.* 2015;372:153–60.

Shear MK, Simon N, Wall M, Zisook S, Neimeyer R, Duan N, et al. Complicated grief and related bereavement issues for DSM-5. *Depression and Anxiety.* 2011;28:103–117.

Stroebe M, Schut H, Finkenauer C. The traumatization of grief? A conceptual framework for understanding the trauma-bereavement interface. *Israel Journal of Psychiatry and Related Sciences.* 2001;38(3–4):185–201.

van der Werff SJA, van den Berg SM, Pannekoek JN, Elzenga BM, van der Wee NJA. Neuroimaging resilience to stress: A review. *Frontiers in Behavioral Neuroscience.* 2013;7(39):1–14.

Zisook S, DeVaul R. Unresolved grief. *The American Journal of Psychoanalysis.* 1985;45(4):370–379.

Zisook S, Iglewicz A, Avanzino J, Maglione J, Glorioso D, Zetumer S, et al. Bereavement: Course, consequences, and care. *Current Psychiatry Reports.* 2014;16(482):1–10.

Chapter 8. The Science of the Wounded Brain

Bejjani BP, Daumier P, Arnulf I, Thivard L, Bonnet AM, Dormont D, et al. Transient acute depression induced by high-frequency deep-brain stimulation. *New England Journal of Medicine.* 1999;340:1476–1480.

Diamond DM, Zoladz PR. Dysfunctional or hyperfunctional? The amygdala in posttraumatic stress disorder is the bull in the evolutionary China shop. *Journal of Neuroscience Research.* 2016; 94:437–444.

Freed PJ, Yanagihara TK, Hirsch J, Mann JJ. Neural mechanisms of grief regulation. *Biological Psychiatry.* 2009;66:33–40.

Gundel H, O'Connor MF, Littrell L, Fort C, Lane RD. Functional neuroanatomy of grief: An fMRI study. *American Journal of Psychiatry.* 2003;160:1946–1953.

Hall M, Irwin M. Physiological indices of functioning in bereavement. In: Stroebe MS, Hansson RO, Stroebe W, Schut H, eds. *Handbook of Bereavement Research: Consequences, Coping, and Care.* Washington, DC: American Psychological Association; 2001: 473–492.

Haq IU, Foote KD, Goodman WG, Wu SS, Sudhyadhom A, Ricciutti N, et al. Smile and laughter induction and intraoperative predictors of response to deep brain stimulation for obsessive compulsive disorder. *Neuroimage.* 2011;54S1:S247-S255.

Holland JM, Rozalski V, Thompson KL, Tiongson RJ, Schatzberg AF, O'Hara R, et al. The unique impact of late-life bereavement and prolonged grief on diurnal cortisol. *Journals of Gerontology. Series B: Psychological Sciences and Social Sciences.* 2013;69(1):4–11.

Lyon AR, Bossone E, Schneider B, Sechtem U, Citro R, Underwood SR, et al. Current state of knowledge on Takotsubo syndrome: A position statement from the task force on Takotsubo syndrome of the Heart Failure Association of the European Society of Cardiology. *European Journal of Heart Failure.* 2016;18:8–27.

Meerwijk EL, Ford JM, Weiss SJ. Brain regions associated with psychological pain: Implications for a neural network and its relationship to physical pain. *Brain Imaging and Behavior.* 2013;7:1–14.

O'Connor MF. Bereavement and the brain: Invitation to a conversation between bereavement researchers and neuroscientists. *Death Studies.* 2005;29:905–922.

O'Connor MF. Immunological and neuroimaging biomarkers of complicated grief. *Dialogues in Clinical Neuroscience.* 2012;14(2):141–148.

O'Connor MF, Irwin MR, Wellisch DK. When grief heats up: Pro-inflammatory cytokines predict regional brain activation. *NeuroImage.* 2009;47:891–896.

Sajeev J, Koshy A, Rajakariar K, Gordon G. Takotsubo cardiomyopathy and transient global amnesia: A shared aetiology. *British Medical Journal Case Reports.* July 14, 2017. doi:10.1136/bcr-2017-219472.

Sharkey SW, Lesser JR, Maron BJ, et al. Cardiology patient page. *Takotsubo (stress) cardiomyopathy.* Circulation 2011;124:e460–2.doi:10.1161/CIRCULA-TIONAHA.111.052662.

Sinha SS. Trauma-induced insomnia: A novel model for trauma and sleep research. *Sleep Medicine Reviews.* 2016;25:74–83.

Williams NR, Okun MS. Deep brain stimulation (DBS) at the interface of neurology and psychiatry. *Journal of Clinical Investigation.* 2013;123(11):4546–4556.

Young LJ, Wang Z. The neurobiology of pair bonding. *Nature Neuroscience.* 2004;7(10):1048–1054.

Chapter 9. Developing Confidence in Managing Grief and Loss

Adler T. The taste of serendipity. *New York Times Magazine.* November 15, 2015.

Arbuckle NW, de Vries B. The long-term effects of later life spousal and parental bereavement on personal functioning. *The Gerontologist.* 1995;35(5):637–647.

Bateson MC. *Composing a Life.* New York: Grove Press; 1989.

Bauer JJ, Bonanno GA. I can, I do, I am: The narrative differentiation of self-efficacy and other self-evaluations while adapting to bereavement. *Journal of Research in Personality.* 2001;35:424–448.

Benight CC, Bandura A. Social cognitive theory of posttraumatic recovery: The role of perceived self-efficacy. *Behaviour Research and Therapy.* 2004;42:1129–1148.

Chan CLW, Ng SM, Ho RTH, Chow AYM. East meets West: Applying Eastern spirituality in clinical practice. *Journal of Clinical Nursing.* 2006;15:822–832.

Christoff K, Irving ZC, Fox KC, Spreng RN, Andrews-Hanna JR. Mind-wandering as spontaneous thought: a dynamic framework. *Nature Reviews Neuroscience*. 2016;17(11):718–731.

Hobson CJ, Kamen J, Szostek J, Nethercut C, Tiedmann J, Wojnarowicz S. Stressful life events: A revision and update of the Social Readjustment Rating Scale. *International Journal of Stress Management*. 1998;5(1):1–23.

Holmes TH, Rahe RH. The Social Readjustment Rating Scale. *Journal of Psychosomatic Research*. 1967;11:213–218.

Isaacson W. *Einstein: His Life and Universe*. New York: Simon and Schuster; 2007.

Klein D. *Travels with Epicurus: A Journey to a Greek Island in Search of a Fulfilled Life*. New York NY: Penguin Group; 2012.

Kobasa SC. Stressful life events, personality and health: an inquiry into hardiness. *Journal of Personality and Social Psychology*. 1979;37(1):1–11.

Linley PA, Joseph S. The human capacity for growth through adversity. *American Psychologist*, 2005;60(3):262–264.

Phillips A. *Becoming Freud*. New Haven: Yale University Press; 2014.

Rilke RM. *Letters to a Young Poet*. New York: Vintage Books; 1986.

Reichl R. *My Kitchen Year: 136 Recipes that Saved My Life*. New York: Penguin Random House; 2015.

Tedeschi RG, Calhoun LG. Posttraumatic growth: Conceptual foundations and empirical evidence. *Psychological Inquiry*. 2004;15(1):1–18.

Tedeschi RG, Calhoun LG. *Trauma & Transformation: Growing in the Aftermath of Suffering*. Thousand Oaks, CA: Sage Publications; 1995.

Utz RL, Lund DA, Caserta MS, deVries B. Perceived self-competency among the recently bereaved. *Journal of Social Work in End-of-Life & Palliative Care*. 2011;7(2–3):173–194.

Woo IMH, Chan CLW, Chow AYM, Ho RTH. Chinese widowers' self-perception of growth: An exploratory study. *Journal of Social Work in End-of-Life & Palliative Care*. 2016;3(4):47–67.

Yalom ID. *Staring at the Sun: Overcoming the Terror of Death*. San Francisco, CA: Jossey-Bass; 2009.

Yalom ID, Lieberman MA. Bereavement and heightened existential awareness. *Psychiatry*. 1991;54:334–345.

Chapter 10. Journaling as a Tool of Emotional Healing

Didion J. *The Year of Magical Thinking*. New York: Alfred Knopf; 2006.

Frisina PG, Borod JC, Lepore SJ. A meta-analysis of the effects of written emotional disclosure on the health outcomes of clinical populations. *The Journal of Nervous and Mental Disease*. 2004;192(9):629–634.

Julavits H. *The Folded Clock: A Diary*. New York: Doubleday; 2015.

Jung C. *Part I: The Archetypes and the Collective Unconscious*. In: Hull RFC, trans. *The Collected Works of C. G. Jung*. Vol. 9. 2nd ed. Princeton, NJ: Princeton University Press; 1968.

McCullough, David. *John Adams.* New York: Simon & Schuster; 2001.

O'Connor M, Nikoletti S, Kristjanson LJ, Loh R, Willcock B. Writing therapy for the bereaved: Evaluation of an intervention. *Journal of Palliative Medicine.* 2003;6(2):195–204.

Pennebaker JW. *Opening Up: The Healing Power of Expressive Emotions.* New York: Guilford Press; 1997.

Pennebaker JW, Beall SK. Confronting a traumatic event: Toward an understanding of inhibition and disease. *Journal of Abnormal Psychology.* 1986;95:274–281.

Pennebaker JW, Mayne TJ, Francis ME. Linguistic predictors of adaptive bereavement. *Journal of Personality and Social Psychology.* 1997;72:863–871.

Petrie KJ, Booth RJ, Pennebaker JW. The immunologic effects of thought suppression. *Journal of Personality and Social Psychology.* 1998;75(5):1264–72.

Petrie KJ, Fontanilla I, Thomas MG, Booth RJ, Pennebaker JW. Effect of written emotional expression on immune function in patients with human immunodeficiency virus infection: A randomized trial. *Psychosomatic Medicine.* 2004;66:272–275.

Ryan, Judith Lingle. Reweaving the self: Creative writing in response to tragedy. *Psychoanalytic Review.* 2009;96(3):529–538.

Spann C. *Poet Healer: Contemporary Poems for Health and Healing.* Sacramento, CA: Sutter's LAMP; 2004.

Zinsser W. *On Writing Well: The Classic Guide to Writing Nonfiction,* 7th Ed. New York: HarperCollins; 2006.

Chapter 11. Nontraditional and Traditional Therapies

Bui E, Nadal-Vicens M, Simon NM. Pharmacological approaches to the treatment of complicated grief: Rationale and a brief review of the literature. *Dialogues in Clinical Neuroscience.* 2012;14(2):149–57.

Chan CLW, Ng SM, Ho RTH, Chow AYM. East meets West: Applying Eastern spirituality in clinical practice. *Journal of Clinical Nursing.* 2006;15:822–832.

Eisma MC, Boelen PA, van den Bout J, Stroebe W, Schut HA, Lancee J, et al. Internet-based exposure and behavioral activation for complicated grief and rumination: A randomized controlled trial. *Behavior Therapy.* 2015;46:729–48.

Isaacson W. *Einstein: His Life and Universe.* New York: Simon and Schuster; 2007.

Jordan JR, Neimeyer RA. Does grief counseling work? *Death Studies.* 2003;27:765–786.

Kogler M, Brandl J, Brandstatter M, Borasio GD, Fegg MJ. Determinants of the effect of existential behavioral therapy for bereaved partners: a qualitative study. *Journal of Palliative Medicine.* 2013;16(11):1410–1416.

Kumar S. Ascending the spiral staircase of grief. In: Kerman M, ed. *Clinical Pearls of Wisdom: 21 Leading Therapists Offer Their Key Insights.* New York: W.W. Norton & Co.; 2010: 118–129.

Lazar SW, Kerr CE, Wasserman RH, Gray JR, Greve DN, Treadway MT, et al. Meditation experience is associated with increased cortical thickness. *Neuroreport.* 2005;16(17):1893–97.

Lewis CS. *A Grief Observed.* New York: HarperCollins; 1994. First published 1961 by N.W. Clerk.

Lutz A, Greischar LL, Rawlings NB, Ricard M, Davidson RJ. Long-term meditators self-induce high-amplitude gamma synchrony during mental practice. *Proceedings of the National Academy of Sciences.* 2004;101(46):16369–16373.

Mohr DC, Lovera J, Brown T, Cohen B, Neylan T, Henry R, et al. A randomized trial of stress management for the prevention of new brain lesions in MS. *Neurology.* 2012;79(5):412–9.

Ogrodniczuk JS, Piper WE, Joyce AS, McCallum M, Rosie JS. NEO-Five factor personality traits as predictors of response to two forms of group psychotherapy. *International Journal of Group Psychotherapy.* 2003;53:4:417–42.

Reynolds CF, Miller MD, Pasternak RE, Frank E, Perel JM, Cornes C, et al. Treatment of bereavement-related major depressive episodes in later life: A controlled study of acute and continuation treatment with nortriptyline and interpersonal psychotherapy. *American Journal of Psychiatry.* 1999;156:202–08.

Roepke AM. Psychosocial interventions and post-traumatic growth: A meta-analysis. *Journal of Consulting and Clinical Psychology.* 2015;83(1):129–42.

Rosenbaum S, Vancampfort D, Steel Z, Newby J, Ward PB, Stubbs B. Physical activity in the treatment of post-traumatic stress disorder: A systematic review and meta-analysis. *Psychiatry Research.* 2015;230:130–136.

Schut HAW, Stroebe MS, van den Bout J, de Keijser J. Intervention for the bereaved: Gender differences in the efficacy of two counselling programmes. *British Journal of Clinical Psychology.* 1997;36:63–72.

Wells RE, Yeh GY, Kerr CE, Wolkin J, Davis RB, Tan Y, et al. Meditation's impact on default mode network and hippocampus in mild cognitive impairment: A pilot study. *Neuroscience Letters.* 2013;556:15–19.

Chapter 12. Emotional Restoration

Kierkegaard S. *Papers and Journals: A Selection.* New York: Penguin Classics; 1996.

Yalom, ID. *Staring at the Sun: Overcoming the Terror of Death.* San Francisco, CA: Jossey-Bass; 2009.

Index